Caregiv Jewish Tradition

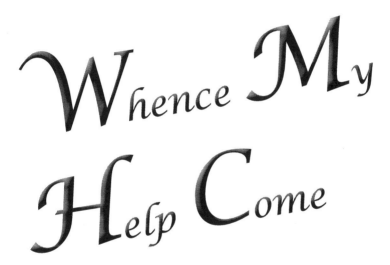

Whence My Help Come

Yisrael Kestenbaum

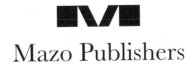

Mazo Publishers

Whence My Help Come: Caregiving in the Jewish Tradition
ISBN 978-1500882839

Text Copyright © 2014 Yisrael Kestenbaum

Contact The Author
Email: ik5769@gmail.com

Published by:
Mazo Publishers
P.O. Box 10474 ~ Jacksonville, FL 32247

Email: mazopublishers@gmail.com
www.mazopublishers.com

When Rabbi Yosef would hear his mother's footsteps, he would say, "Let me rise before the Divine presence that is passing."
Talmud Kiddushin 31b

To my mother, Hannah Kestenbaum...

Like the *Shekhina*, she has always provided loving protection and care for her children, grandchildren and great-grandchildren.

Table of Contents

About The Author

Yisrael Kestenbaum had a long career as a pastoral educator and chaplain. He has *semicha* (rabbinic ordination) from the Ner Israel Rabbinical College in Baltimore and holds two Masters Degrees, one in Philosophy, and one in Education from the University of Western Ontario.

Kestenbaum is an avid writer, and authors a weekly blog, *The Torah and the Self.* He has also published many articles in the field of pastoral care.

Kestenbaum learns Torah and serves as Events Coordinator for the Rotenberg Center for Jewish Psychology in Jerusalem.

Author's Preface

The content of this book was scheduled for publication now more than seven years ago. I was then the Director of The Jewish Institute for Pastoral Care at The Health-Care Chaplaincy in New York. My life fell apart after pleading guilty to an offense, and the book got buried.

While my crime had no victim and the only ones hurt by my actions, in the end, were the ones I loved most and who indeed loved me, I realize that I made a serious error in judgment. I have spent the intervening years doing a heartfelt and sober *teshuva*.

My beloved wife, Pamela, who stood with me and encouraged me through this process tragically passed away of cancer now two years ago. I live in Jerusalem with our daughter Bess. I no longer practice pastoral care professionally nor function as a rabbi. I study Torah and devote my life to the service of Hashem and doing *hesed*.

While my experience has taught me that much that is lost is irretrievable, it has also taught me that what can be salvaged should not be tossed away. It is in that spirit, and with my sentence completed, that I decided to publish this book. I do not publish as a means to any personal agenda, but rather to share what I learned in my years of practicing and teaching pastoral care with Jewish caregivers, who may learn something that will help them in their service to others.

My own experience over these last years has only served to make me more sensitive to the world of the marginalized and the hurting. I hope releasing the book may enhance our compassion and understanding of their plight.

May G-d in His great compassion bring healing to all who have been wounded. May He who I most offended see this book as a personal expression of atonement.

Humbly,
Yisrael Kestenbaum
June 2009

Acknowledgements

There are many acknowledgements of thanks I offer on completing this manuscript and finally bringing it to life.

I am grateful to Dr. Jack Berezov formerly of the Jewish Institute for Pastoral Care of the HealthCare Chaplaincy who worked with me to ready the text.

I thank Rabbis Bunny Friedman and Dannel Schwartz of the Michigan Board of Rabbis who many years ago envisioned this project as a means to make rabbis comfortable with an approach to caregiving that often felt foreign.

I appreciate the encouragement of Leonard Kestenbaum, my uncle, who believed that the book was important and should come to life even if delayed.

I thank my son Avi for his belief in my gifts as a parent and teacher.

Thanks to my brother Josh for his daily phone call to ask how I and my work was progressing.

And to Bess, who I now raise alone, who has been my life's joy and for making each day a gift.

I am indebted to the men and women I was privileged to care for and to my students whose lives and struggles brought me to wisdom. Through their journeys, I have been enlivened. It is their truths I am privileged to reveal.

It saddens me that *Whence My Help Come: Caregiving in the Jewish Tradition* will be released now near two years since the passing of my beloved wife Pamela, herself a superb caregiver and source of inspiration to me. Her journey of courage and struggle challenges me each day to live with meaning. I miss her and yet I feel her presence always. May the book's release be a source of *nachas* for her in the world eternal.

If I could reduce all of what I know about caregiving, all of this book, to one thought, even as Hillel did for all of Judaism, in the famous story of the Talmud, I would say, "to provide spiritual care is not to give to another but to receive from them. That is the central truth. The rest is all commentary. Go and learn!"

YK

Introduction

She lay in the bed, the image of Sleeping Beauty. Her blond hair spread across the pillow. Her skin was white and smooth. She looked peaceful amidst the covers and in the soft décor of her room. Only she wasn't sleeping. She was not yet twenty-one. And she was dead.

Naomi had lost her struggle against cancer. She had fought valiantly, her family by her side. Now they sat around her bed. Her father, swaying as if in prayer, every so often gave out a painful whimper. Her mother sat stoically, red-eyed, both from exhaustion and from tears. Her many brothers and sisters paid silent homage to their sibling, now gone. Through Naomi's illness, they insisted she never lose her place in the life of the family. Even her brother's wedding ceremony was replayed in the home dining room so Naomi could hear the service from her upstairs bedroom.

When I joined the community to serve as rabbi six months earlier, Naomi's illness was already pretty far advanced. Not having been there from the beginning, I did not know how to easily enter the drama. I visited Naomi when she was in the hospital. I tried to be supportive of her family. But in truth, I was afraid to ask about her prognosis, and I guess no one wanted to tell. I was a young rabbi thrust into a situation I was unprepared to handle.

But now Naomi was dead. And I needed to be with the family. I went to the house and entered the scene I described above. The beautiful princess was dead in her bed. The family – father, mother and siblings – were sitting around in an awesome silence, punctuated by the occasional sob. What could I say? What could I do?

I found a chair. I took a seat with the mourners. I knew something needed to happen. The funeral home needed to be called, arrangements made, perhaps some good-byes, some closure. We could not stay here forever. But the setting was larger than me. And I, too, was captured within its poignancy and power. Time was frozen. I had no words. I had little sense of self. Moments passed. No one moved. I was as immobile as Naomi's family. It felt as if we sat there for hours.

Over the years that have elapsed since that sad yet stirring event, I have often thought that if the family physician had not walked in and, in his own matter-of-fact way, moved the family along, we might still be sitting by Naomi's bedside.

I surmise that every rabbi in his or her professional career has a story not unlike my experience at the bedside with Naomi and her family. To be authentic in this work is to have moments of feeling totally overwhelmed by the awesome circumstances we confront. This book is the product of a journey I made in the aftermath of my deathbed care with Naomi and other caregiving moments, similar moments, where I knew I wanted to provide a healing presence but didn't know how.

This book is about giving those who provide spiritual care, both rabbis and others motivated to serve as instruments of healing, the conceptual models and practical tools to do the holy work of *hesed*, loving-kindness. It is one thing to have a good heart. It is another to have the sophistication to exercise one's goodness of heart in constructive interventions to promote healing for others in their times of suffering.

My own journey led me to take Clinical Pastoral Education (CPE) while I served the congregation where Naomi's family belonged. I learned in CPE the discipline of care; how one needs to respect the other even before attempting to help. I learned about relationships, about the dynamics of families, about suffering, about illness and loss. One unit of CPE followed another. I grew in my skills and in my ability to define my role as caregiver in the context of suffering.

Most of all, I learned about myself. I learned to recognize my strengths and weaknesses that I might better enter in healing re-lationships to mitigate the aloneness and help the hurting other feel the love of the Divine. My own journey as a rabbi occurred in a CPE world devoid of Jews. All my supervisors were Christian. All my peer groups consisted of clergy from other faiths. The prin-ciples taught felt valid and useful. The idioms and paradigms used to teach them felt foreign.

When I was certified as a supervisor of Clinical Pastoral Educa-tion by the American Association for Clinical Pastoral Education (ACPE), I was determined to recast what I learned into the lan-guage and values of the Jewish tradition. Over the better part of a decade, I have educated rabbis, Jewish seminarians, and Jewish lay leaders in CPE. My students have challenged me to integrate the truths inherent in the literature of pastoral care with the core concepts of Judaism. This book does just that. It is indeed a Jewish companion to Clinical Pastoral Education. More, it challenges the Jewish caregiver from the very sources of his/her own tradition to conceptual and practical competence.

The rabbis taught that "there is no wisdom like that born out of the living challenge." This book presents both a theology of caregiving and the guidelines for interventions. The early chapters concentrate on presenting a model for the work of *hesed*. In Chap-ter One, we explicate the place of *hesed* in the constellation of Jewish values. In Chapters Two and Three, we explore the essential realities of suffering and its remediation. Chapter Four invites the rabbi in particular to consider the unique and different challenges he/she is called upon to confront in the role of caregiving in con-trast to the teaching role. In Chapter Five, the caregiver is invited to see his/her place in the triad of God, the suffering others and as the agent of help.

The later chapters of the book confront the work of caregiv-ing in its more particular settings. The chapter on spiritual assess-ment utilizes verbatim snippets and Hassidic stories to create a framework for diagnosis and intervention. In Chapter Seven, we consider the place of prayer and its utilization as an instrument for healing. Chapters Eight, Nine and Ten explore the pastoral issues of shame, grief and loss, and hope and despair respectively. In each instance, the particular pastoral issue is examined from the conceptual and practical vantage points, and in each instance, we reference traditional Jewish sources.

Finally, the book concludes with a chapter "Knowing Thyself." It asks the question all caregivers must confront: "What is there for me in this?" It also helps put the self-need common to all caregivers in potentially healing perspective.

So with all that you may well ask, "Will this book make me a good caregiver?" Sorry to say, just as a book on parenting will not turn the new father or mother into a good parent, this book will not make you a good caregiver. No matter how well it is written or how relevant its content, to become proficient in a work involving relationships you need more than a book offering cognitive insight. You need experience. You need practice. This book will teach you why and tell you how. But it remains a conceptual reference point. It is for you to engage in the real life work of caregiving and see how it matches and differs from what you expected about yourself, about the other, and about suffering.

If I ask myself, Had I read a book like this, would I have been better able to engage Naomi's family around her death bed?, I cannot honestly say "yes." Even now, some twenty years later, reflecting on what I did at the bedside that day, I remain unsure. What this book does is give a language and perspective to the questions I had then, but could not frame, of what indeed was my role and responsibility. It offers me the tools to evaluate my professional work. It provides a discipline for *hesed* through which assessment of self and others become possible.

The book is best used in concert with clinical opportunities to practice providing spiritual care. It is ideal as a companion to CPE, and it was written with my students in mind. Better still, the book should be used in concert with both clinical practice and supervision. It provides the concepts and the clinical models to foster a dialogue between the students of spiritual care and their supervisors by which to reflect on their work.

Caregiving
in the Jewish Tradition

Chapter 1
Whence Will My Help Come...

T he desire to help is a core human emotion. Extending oneself to another is as much a need as an act of beneficence. We are helpers. When the Jewish Family Service of the Jewish community in which I served as a rabbi did a survey to assess the needs of the aging and how the agency might improve its programming to better address those needs, it discovered that more of those surveyed were interested in how they could help others than in how they could be helped. When we help others, we experience our value. Our life has meaning. We claim our place in society and feel affirmed. When we are unable to find a helping context, our sense of value is compromised. We doubt our usefulness. We often surrender to a despair born out of a lack of life meaning.

The centrality of helping to the quality of life should not surprise us as Jews. The Psalmist tells us "...I have fashioned a world of kindness".[1] In his classic *The Way of God*, Rabbi Moshe Chaim Luzzatto explained that the whole of creation only came to be so that God could bestow God's kindness on another. God, too, has the desire to help. It was out of this desire and God's yearning to provide "good" to another that God made the world and formed human beings in God's image to be the objects of God's desire and claim the "good" God wants for them.[2]

---

1. Psalms 89:3

2. Moshe Chaim Luzzatto, translated and annotated by Aryeh Kaplan, *Derech Hashem, The Way of God* (Jerusalem & New York: Feldheim 1997), Part 1, 2:1

Part of our being fashioned in God's image seems to be our need to help. When Adam, the first human, is placed in the Garden of Eden, he has everything save one. All the beauty, all the variety, all the splendor is still insufficient. The Torah says "…and for man he did not find a helpmate opposite him".[3] When God does in fact create Eve, she is brought to Adam not for the purpose of being a sexual partner or even to mitigate his loneliness as a companion. Rather, Eve is to be for Adam a "helpmate opposite him." It is the mutual relationship of helping that needs to be addressed in the creation of Eve. No paradise can be complete if a helping relationship is not part of it.

But if the desire to help is so inextricably linked to who we are and so central to our nature, we would do well to wonder why it is so difficult to help successfully. Sure, it seems a relatively simple gesture to deposit a dollar bill in the container for the homeless. It's not hard to write a check to a charitable institution or even to help a stranger across the street. Yet the helping situations that are most intimate and most important to our lives are infinitely more complex. When we try to help the people we love most, we often not only fail, we engender a reactivity that often leaves us stunned. Let me cite the following vignette.

Debbie, a high-school junior, bursts through the door of her house after school and tells her mother that her boyfriend of six months has just broken up with her so he can date other girls. Debbie is distraught and weeping. Through her tears, she tells her mother that she feels ugly, that she hates her former boyfriend, that she also loves him, that she wants to die.

Debbie's mother, who has not been very fond of the boy-friend, is relieved that the relationship is over, but she is disturbed to see her daughter so obviously heartbroken and unhappy. Debbie is inconsolable as her mother tries to cheer her by telling her how pretty she is and how she will attract new boyfriends. She also tells Debbie that she never really

---

3. Genesis 2:20

liked the boyfriend but didn't say anything while they were dating because Debbie cared for him so much. The more her mother talks, the more upset Debbie becomes.

"You don't understand me!" Debbie screams. "Leave me alone! I don't want to talk to you! You don't understand anything!"

Debbie withdraws and refuses to talk to her mother at all. She is miserable and her mother feels terrible.[4]

In each of our lives, scenes like the above are repeated over and over. A wife tries to help her husband by sharing some useful advice only to receive a taciturn remark in response. Parents who want only to get their children through a difficult time find themselves thwarted and rebuffed at every turn. If we were to examine instances of family discord and argument closely, we would find so many of the most intense flare-ups occur precisely when one family member thought he/she was going to help the other. It is in reaction to helping gestures that many of the painful conflicts erupt. Not only does the person we seek to help reject our effort forcefully, as Debbie did in our example, we become defensive in response. We feel outraged that our good intentions get maligned. The conflict escalates until we might not even remember the helping gesture with which the struggle began.

What goes wrong? Surely the situation warrants help. Our desire was founded in love. How does that which feels so right turn so wrong?

Rachel Naomi Remen in a short and poignant piece entitled *In the Service of Life* captured a truth vital to understanding helping relationships, whether they be personal or out of the professional role of caregiving. She distinguished what she referred to as "helping" and "fixing" from the sacred call to "service." She noted in the article that the problem of helping is that it is always based on an inequality. "It is not a relationship between equals.

---

4. Jean Baker Miller and Irene Pierce Stiver, *The Healing Connection: How Women Form Relationships in Therapy and in Life* (Boston: Beacon Press, 1997), p 10

When you help you use you use your own strength to help those of lesser strength....People feel this inequality. When we help we may inadvertently take away from people more than we could ever give them, we may diminish their self-esteem, their sense of worth, integrity and wholeness."[5]

She noted that helping incurs debt. "When you help someone they owe you one." Remen went on to reflect critically on the role of fixing as well. When we fix someone, we see them as broken. We fix from a distance. We judge their limitations and seek to make a correction. Here, too, there is inequality in the relationship, an inequality of expertise that can easily become a moral distance.

In the vignette cited above, Debbie's mother is engaged in the work of fixing Debbie. She made an effort to right Debbie's erroneous perspective in order to relieve her hurt. She tried to help Debbie by lending her own strength and wisdom to shore up Debbie's shattered self-esteem. While nothing Debbie's mother said was untrue, it only exacerbated Debbie's sense of inadequacy. Remen noted for herself, "With 40 years of chronic illness I have been helped by many people and fixed by a great many others who did not recognize my wholeness. All that fixing and helping left me wounded in some important and fundamental ways."[6] The context in caregiving is as vital as the content. If the context says, "You are weak, broken, stupid, silly, etc.", it does not matter how good the content of our helping message, it will not only fail to be heard, it will often engender a hostile response.

Let's reflect for a moment on the darker side of our desire to help. While all that we explored in the first part of this chapter on the centrality of helping to the *raison d'être* for the world's existence and the character of humankind is true, it does not mean that all our efforts to help emerge from a sacred place. When we see someone struggling, our impulse to help has two sources. Out of the holy dimension the urge to help another emerges from the awareness that the other's struggle is our struggle, too. We are all

---

5. Rachel Naomi Remen, *In the Service of Life* in Noetic Science Review (Spring 1996)

6. Ibid

one. The other's story is our story. As Jews, we oft times repeat the refrain of our essential unity. When one Jew suffers all are affected. The well-being of each individual is vital to the well-being of the community. At a more inclusive level, much the same can be said to be true of our relationship to humanity as a whole.

The Talmud teaches "to save a single life is to save the whole world."[7] When we help another because we experience his/her predicament as ours, the helping act builds community, engenders love, and fosters healing. It is this kind of helping that Remen refers to as service. For Remen, service is always a relationship between equals. We serve with all of our experiences, our limitations, our wounds, even our darkness can serve. Service is always about "we" even if one member of the "we" relationship is more active in response to the circumstances.

The darker side of helping emerges out of other emotions. Dorothy Soelle in her classic work *Suffering* presented a compelling account of the human response to suffering as emanating from the desire to distance ourselves from the wounded other.[8] Like its more noble form, the darker response to suffering begins with an identification with the struggling. But unlike the sacred response to the person struggling, in its darker imitations our response is to protect ourselves from being affected by the circumstances. We use helping as a way to distance ourselves from the other person, so as to stand above him/her in order to feel safe. We give advice precisely so we don't have to feel the we-ness with its attendant vulnerability. We share wisdom and counsel, precisely to keep problems in the other person's yard. When we are told someone has died, our most immediate response is a question. "How old was she?" The unconscious root of the query is to get an answer than will make us feel safe. If she was 87, then we don't have to worry when we are 53. When someone has cancer, our first impulse is to find a cause: "Did he smoke?" Here, too, if we can identify a reason we don't have to feel anxious that the disease will affect us as well. The urge to separate ourselves from the suffering of another is as instinctual

---

7. Sanhedrin 37a

8. Dorothy Soelle, *Suffering* (Philadelphia: Fortress Press, 1975)

as the urge to offer help.

The desire to insulate ourselves from the suffering of another has its roots in our perceived similarity. It is because we feel so close that we respond by engendering distance. The closer we are, the more the problem hits home, the more likely we will be to respond with the kind of help born out of a desire to demonstrate concern and yet engender for us a sense of safety.

The examples we can cite are everyday and familiar. The husband comes home from work. His wife has had a hard day. She struggled with the school over a discipline problem with one of their children. The wife tells the husband of her distress, of the impasse she has reached with both the teacher and their child. The husband hears his wife's sense of frustration and powerlessness. He needs to respond. He could comfort his wife, join her in experiencing her struggle and become a partner with her in both her shame and anger. Or he could distance himself by giving his wife a suggestion of how she could handle the problem, what she should tell the teacher or say to their child. Sadly, in most instances the husband will choose the latter form of response. He will feel anxious lest his wife's indecisiveness becomes more of a problem for him and the family. Rather than see the issue as concerning his child and the school, he will see the problem as his wife's limitations and respond to her brokenness with either a fixing or helping intervention.

Is it any wonder men and women in relationships often feel unheard and diminished. Yet surprisingly those closest to them will often be the last to know. They will claim surprise and bewilderment inasmuch as they always saw themselves as ready and committed to help.

Professional caregivers often face similar challenges. The rabbi or chaplain visiting a patient or congregant in the hospital will most frequently respond to a presentation of problems by offering advice, giving a suggestion, or volunteering a strategy. Caregivers need to ask themselves what is motivating the response. In most cases, the suggestions come not because the patient/congregant solicited them. On the contrary, the patient/congregant in most cases simply shared his/her struggle. The helping gestures more typically emerge out of the need of the caregiver who simply cannot tolerate being intimate with one suffering without distancing him/herself with a piece of advice, a suggestion or a new strategy. The context of the message is in conflict with the content. While the content says, "I want to help you," the context says, "Keep your problems to yourself." In the very guise of the helping relationship, what is occurring is the diminishment of the patient/congregant. As Remen said about her own experience, this style of helping and fixing leaves the cared for "wounded in some important and fundamental ways." If that is true of her story with secular caregivers of whom she wrote, how much more serious the impact if the caregiver is a rabbi or chaplain and in fact representing both the faith community and the Divine.

So how do we recognize if our response is coming from the sacred dimension of the desire to help within or from its not only less holy but frequently harmful counterpart? Rabbi Edwin Friedman once remarked that the way he knew the appropriate intervention to make in a therapeutic relationship was to consider his impulsive response and then do the opposite. In his wisdom, he realized that his natural reaction would be a response to his own anxiety, his desire to distance himself from the story of the other so as to feel safe from the consequences. To reveal the real direction caregiving requires, we need to do more than pass on our impulsive first response. We need to study the source of our anxiety. In the end, the response we would make were we able to suspend our anxiety is the true and relational one.

To help we need to first be disciplined. Even before reaching out to another, we need to become comfortable in the presence of another's hurt. The key truth here is that helping is not teaching. It is not about having wisdom, insight or perspective to bear on the situation. Nor is helping at its deepest level about doing for another. Maimonides already made clear in his discussion of the eight stages of charity that the highest level of charity is a charitable act that permits the other person to live without dependency.[9] If helping another to remain independent, self-reliant, and feeling

---

9. Maimonides, Hilchot Matnot Aneyem, 10:7

whole is the highest goal of a charitable monetary gift, how much more so would a gift of person require similar aspiration? In helping another, we want not simply to solve the other person's problem but to help him/her feel enabled to meet life's challenges, feel confident, restore his/her trust in the world as a place that can be inhabited without fear. Only a response born out of relationship can do that. Only a helping gesture emerging from a non-anxious, patient, expression of love can realize that end.

Love is the operative dynamic in all our efforts to help. Maimonides understood the responsibility to provide care as emanating from the Torah's call of "Love thy neighbor as thyself"[10].[11] The specific *mitzvot*, such as visiting the sick, comforting the mourner, and so on, are rabbinic imperatives that are gleaned from the Torah's challenge to love our neighbor. To help someone, we need to first love him/her. We must feel his/her heartache, disappointment, and need. It is not enough to understand the problem in its complexity and have the right answer. We need to feel with the hurting person. Loving the patient/congregant as a person with his/her problems will lead us to respond in ways that enhance self-esteem and encourage hope, not only about the problematic situation but about the person's own capacity to deal with it.

In the very early story of the Garden of Eden discussed above, Eve is brought to Adam so they could live in a helping relationship. The Torah's use of term is fascinating. Eve was created to be what literally translates as "a helpmate opposite him".[12] The term "opposite" has engendered much commentary among rabbinic scholars. They wonder, if she is a "helpmate," how can she be "opposite" (if opposite implies adversary). In light of our discussion, the challenges for Adam and Eve to live as opposites in the helping relationship seem profoundly clear. Yes, Adam and Eve were brought together so that each could express their instinctive need to help. To be made in the image of God means very much to want to bestow kindness on another even as God desires to do kindness.

10. Leviticus 19:18

11. Maimonides, Hilchot Avel, 14:1

12. Genesis 2:18

But the help of God is not the help of humans. When God helps, it is the help of the Infinite One for God's creations. There does indeed accrue an indebtedness. We are God's humble servants. Our life is an expression of appreciations for gifts received and not yet earned. God is not our equal. God is our Sovereign, our Creator. In relationship to God's love for us we feel a gratitude that leads to exaltation.

Adam and Eve while expressing their love toward each other in helping acts need to find another way. Their expressions of care must not be from the "one-up" position. Their care must not engender indebtedness or serve to cause an imbalance. Adam and Eve must become helpmates opposite each other, that is, on the same level, equals, even in moments when one is providing an act of help to the other. It is for this very reason that Eve was not created separate from Adam and at the same time as him in the story of Creation. Making Eve after Adam and from him meant they were essentially one. Adam and Eve may inhabit two bodies and occupy separate space but they share the common genetic makeup. Eve was formed from Adam's rib. That truth makes it wholly inappropriate for Adam to help Eve from a superior position of from the distance of an other. They are one. Eve's issues are Adam's as well and vice versa. They are, at the most elemental level, of one source. In extending care for each other, they are helping themselves. The hurt of the one endangers both. The wellness of each is essential to the other. While lifting one's eyes toward heaven may well be the Psalmist's image for help from the Divine, the help we receive from our human brothers and sisters need be eyes directed at the one opposite us. And if perchance in our moment of needing help we feel below the one who may indeed help us, it becomes their job to get down in order to become opposite, that is, on the same level as we who need help.

The measure of the act of helping that has its source in the sacred can be taken in the feelings we who help are left with after our helping gesture. When we help because we love, we feel a sense of closeness to the one helped. We know a holiness born out of a sacred intimacy, the sharing with another in a community of authentic struggle. We are full of the spirit of the Divine evident when a holy I-Thou encounter has occurred. Helping has the God infused spirituality we often expect to find in prayer, only now rather than reflect the God-human meeting, it is in the encounter of two mortals fused with the spirit of God who meet each other in their mutual striving. In the less noble expression of help, when our gesture emanates from our own anxiety and distance, the satisfaction we feel belongs to the ego. We applaud ourselves for our heroics, our wisdom, our generosity. We may get a quick rush of self-congratulation, but it hardly lasts beyond the next frustration. The satisfaction is ultimately empty, and we require constant new helping heroics to sustain our sense of self-validation and ongoing meaning. The gift of helping through love and relationship is that in its wake we are left with new community. It is not what we have done but what we are a part of. In our belonging to the other, and indeed to all others, we have transcendent meaning and value. We remain forever a part of the drama of life and the story of our people.

In the remaining chapters of this book, we will explore in great depth the discipline we will need in order to help as a sacred act. We will study the self as much as the other, for only in our openness to both can an authentic relationship be established. To the extent we as helpers learn from the act of care, we can do more than bring a blessing to the world, great as that healing act would be. We can attach ourselves to our faith and our people so as to guarantee our sense of meaning through time. In helping we shatter the boundaries that limit us in time and space. We open up the window to eternity.

Chapter 2
The Dynamics of Suffering

The Sheloh, Rabbi Isaiah Horwitz, author of *Sh'nei Luchos Habris*, observed, "There is no moment without its torment. There is no hour that is not sour. There is no day without dismay..."[1] Indeed, Jewish tradition has long recognized that suffering is not an anomaly to life but very much a large component of life's makeup. When Adam and Eve are banished from the Garden of Eden, they are promised struggle. The rest of the Torah in many ways can be seen as the fulfillment of that promise.

Every righteous person, from Abraham to Moses, experiences heartache and disappointment. In Ecclesiastes, Solomon wrote of man, "Also all his days are vexation and pain".[2] Job says "Man is born to struggle – of few days and full of trouble".[3] Jacob, our great patriarch, said to Pharaoh: "Few and bad have been the days of my life".[4] To read the story of King David is to understand the suffering he expresses in the Psalms, for who could endure the betrayal and unfairness of his life and not complain?

Caregiving is a response to suffering. It is not an answer to it. We cannot pretend suffering is avoidable or easily transformed. Suffering is real, constant and inextricable from life. The first discipline a caregiver needs to accept is that he/she is not God, and cannot change the nature of the world's circumstances. Even if

1. Sheloh 2:138a
2. Ecclesiastes 2:23
3. Job 10:1
4. Genesis 47:9

the caregiver could by dint of some brilliant or imaginative inter-vention relieve the sufferer from his/her current predicament, it would be temporary at best. There is no ultimate escape from life's companion. Suffering is our destiny in this material world. In the *mitzvot* of caring, we are challenged to accept that reality for our-selves and others, that we might build a caring community.

I say for ourselves and others, because until we are ready to face the sad and painful truth that we do and will suffer, we will continue to avoid experiencing it in others. When students are seeking ad-mission into Clinical Pastoral Education programs, the premier for-mat for learning how to provide spiritual care, they are asked about their own journey: "What have you struggled with?" "Where are your life's disappointments?" Not uncommonly, the students, often young, filled with their sense of mission, will look dumbfounded in response. They wonder the purpose of the query.

But in reality to the extent that we deny our own suffering and struggle we will be unavailable to accept another's. We will for-ever seek to make their situations an accident of circumstances, something to be remedied, like a bad cold. It is only when we can honestly claim our own hurts for the truths that they are, as much a part of our selves as our strengths and our talents, that the pos-sibility exists that we can become meaningful healing presences in the lives of others.

It would be useful here to distinguish between suffering and pain. When we speak of pain we are describing a neurological phe-nomenon. It is measurable and predictable. For the most part, our pain is causally related to the stimuli. Its presence can be used di-agnostically to reveal some physiological problem and/or malfunc-tion. Suffering is the individual person's response to his/her pain, the meaning he/she gives it, the interpretation it has for him/her in the context of his/her life. The same circumstances will produce totally different experiences of suffering for different people in light of their different approaches to life. Healing pain, while neuro-logically akin to the pain of woundedness, will be experienced as much more bearable. Pain that has meaning for a person engen-ders much less suffering than pain perceived as devoid of meaning.

Two women giving birth, one to a stillborn, the other to a live child, will undergo similar physiological experiences. Their pain if measured might be very much alike. Yet we would expect the mother of the stillborn to suffer to a far greater degree with every contraction than her counterpart anticipating the arrival of her desired and alive child.

It has become quite the agenda in medical institutions today to make pain treatment a focus of care. Palliative care has as one of its primary goals to help patients manage the painful consequences of their chronic conditions. In some institutions I have seen signs with pain written in the midst of a circle and a line running through it expressing the message "no pain here." What's often not understood is that the issues that cause difficulty for most of the ill and compromised is suffering, not pain. No amount of medication will relieve suffering unless it numbs the person's consciousness. Suffering has as its causes a lack of meaning, a purposelessness, fear, loneliness, self-loathing, a diminished sense of value. These are not the kind of issues that get medicated away. They require human responses and healing relationships.

Physicians respond to physiological malfunctioning. They treat the pain associated with that malfunction as well. Their goal is to promote cure. Caregivers respond to the emotional and spiritual issues around life's challenges. They offer a response to suffering. Their goal is healing. Life need not always have pain. Science can see to that. But life will always have suffering. To care is to live with another in that suffering and promote the possibility for healing.

What is the essential ingredient of suffering? In what lies its core reality? If we look to the tradition, we find that suffering in its deepest level is founded in a sense of estrangement. When Adam and Eve sin, their core punishment is banishment from the Garden. Cain upon killing his brother Abel is compelled to wander. Israel's punishment for its sinfulness is *Galut*, exile, estrangement from their land. For many personal sins of serious consequences, the punishment is *Koret*, being cut off. Whatever its practical implications, its meaning is that the sinner is to suffer the hurt of estrangement. At the deepest metaphysical level, estrangement is the existential suffering of life. Tradition sees this world as the necessary separation from our spiritual source in order ultimately to return. The Midrash sees the soul as banished from heaven against its will.[5] Ramchal explains this banishment as a way to invite us to earn our place in the presence of the Divine, so that the pleasure we will know we will feel belongs to us and is no accidental gift.[6] Ironically, even in heaven we can feel estranged if our relationship to God's blessing does not feel earned.

Truth be told, all living is suffering because of the reality that the soul mourns for its home. We feel ourselves existentially alone, separated from the unity we crave and require. Every comfort from the bosom of our mother to the intimacy we share with our spouse is but a shadow of the truer unconditional union with our life's source that we long for. When Adam and Eve ate from the forbidden fruit, they became not only knowing of good and evil, they knew that they knew. They had a level of self-consciousness previously unavailable to them. In that knowing of their knowing, they became frighteningly aware of their individuality and aloneness. They became for the first time afraid. The human response ever since has been to flee that consciousness.

A Zen master was once asked, "What is the greatest miracle?" He replied, "Here I sit alone with myself." Indeed, to sit alone with oneself, fully conscious of one's absolute existential and vulnerable "I," is terrifying. We spend our life insulating ourselves from that awareness. Our careers, our avocations, our frantic resolve to be "doing" something as if just "being" would threaten us emerges out of the need to avoid feeling the nakedness of our aloneness. In this state of consciousness, the first humans needed to be placed outside the Garden. Simply existing in the presence of God yet separated from God, while now fully mortal, was a suffering Adam and Eve would not be able to endure. In our post-Garden world of "doing," we are forever able to distract ourselves from the

<hr>

5. Tanchuma, Pikudei

6. Moshe Chaim Luzzatto, translated and annotated by Aryeh Kaplan, *Derech Hashem, The Way of God* (Jerusalem & New York: Feldheim 1997), Part 1, 2:2

awareness of our estrangement from the Divine and ultimately from our deepest and purest selves.

It is in response to this deep and unavoidable truth that we build families and communities. In its healthiest sense, we do so, not to run away from our individual consciousness, but to give us the courage to live conscious and alert. To become the "whole" person God wills us to be, we need to be conscious. We need to not only do the *mitzvot*, we need to understand our motives and refine our intentions. As the Medrash teaches, "Does the Holy One Blessed Be He really care whether we slaughter (the animal) from the front of the neck or the back? Rather the *mitzvot* we're given to shape the character of (God's) creations."[7] Indeed, *mitzvot* are designed to help us develop our character.

Refinement of character calls for self-awareness, consciousness, being alone with ourselves. Sharing life with others helps us to live with our individuality. Not that it makes us any less alone. Just that we have other alone people with us in our terror that we might persevere in our mission and live out this destiny with meaning.

The relationship between suffering and consciousness helps to explain why those who are sick and/or experiencing life on the margins feel a deep sense of suffering. For illness makes one acutely conscious of one's "I." When one is sick he/she is aware of his/her individuality in all its ramifications. The illness forces the person to get off the merry-go-round of life and to face the existential limitations that are part of his/her makeup. It is not that the sick and marginalized are that different in their predicament from us. After all, we are all alone and vulnerable and at all times. We are all separated from the unity we most need with the Divine. We are all in *Galut* and estranged. Rather it is that sickness forces us inward. We cannot, when sick, escape the sad truth of our condition. In sickness we become conscious to our existential plight. And so we suffer, not our suffering alone, but the suffering of what it means to be human.

The Talmud teaches that the *Shekhina* is above the head of the

---

7. Tanchuma, Shmini

sick, present in the room in times of illness.[8] The remark is more
than metaphor. It has *halachic* implications. One can pray at the
sickbed in any language without concern that it will lose effectiveness, because the *Shekhina* is present in the room and prayer there
is more easily efficacious. We might well wonder what draws the
Shekhina to the sickbed. The sick person him/herself rarely feels it.
On the contrary, in illness one typically experiences God's absence.
As King David exclaimed in his time of suffering, "My God, My
God, Why has Thou forsaken me?"[9] Nor is the *Shekhina* there to
heal in as much as she remains present even when no recovery is
evident.

May I suggest, in light of our conversation, that the *Shekhina* is
present at the bed of the sick because there she finds a companion in the *Galut*. Our tradition has long taught that when Israel
went into *Galut* the *Shekhina* went with them.[10] She is separated
from her source in the *Ein Sof*, the Infinite One, even as Israel is
separated from the land. Where would the *Shekhina* find a place in
the *Galut* if not at the bedside of the sick who, in their heightened
consciousness, suffer the experience of *Galut* and estrangement?
At the bedside the *Shekhina* finds a partner for her own suffering.
The authenticity of the estrangement experience is lived out here
as nowhere else. The *Shekhina* in the sick room finds a community
of the alone with the suffering sick.

But enough now of theological reflection. Let us explore more
explicitly the nature of the suffering of the sick. If we examine the
particulars of the estrangement we can comprehend it at three different levels, with increasing dimensions of severity. The first layer
of estrangement experienced by the sick is a societal estrangement.
When one becomes ill, one is separated from the society he/she
participated in and estranged from his/her social role. In sickness
one cannot go to work, or if he/she does he/she cannot function in
the same way as before. The ill are typically homebound, unable
to play golf with friends, participate in synagogue life, attend

8. BT Nedarim 40a
9. Psalms 22:2
10. BT Megillah 29a

lectures, lead committees, share the traditional morning coffee with the regulars. When one is sick, one's place in the community is absent. He/she no longer occupies his/her seat on the train. His/her place in shul goes vacant or to another. One feels a sense of loss and disconnectedness from the social fabric so much a part of one's sense of who one is.

In the social estrangement, the sick wonder who they are now, separated from the place they have had in community. Once they knew they were esteemed, perhaps a physician or a teacher. Now every nurse that is half their age walks into their room unannounced and calls them "Honey." Separated from their job and place of influence, they have taken on a new identity, that of "patient." It is a role they don't know, confusing and diminishing. Once they had power. People listened and treated them as valued. Now they feel abandoned by a society who merely patronizes its flawed members. The social suffering they experience is akin to that of the leper, ostracized, stripped of dignity. True, the healthy do not perceive their way of engagement as offensive and pernicious. But it is not their intent that we are concerned with here. It is the experience of the ill. And willy-nilly the ill feel the effects of their illness acutely as one of societal estrangement. In entering hospitals, wearing gowns, assuming the role of patient, the experience of estrangement is cause for suffering made only more profound by the fact that it is expressed mostly in silence. For after all, who really is there for them to blame?

The second layer of estrangement affects the sick in relationship to their families. The mother who becomes ill is dealing with more than the issues of her health. She may feel compromised in her role as provider of the family meals, source for the family hospitality, agent for intra-family understanding. In her compromised state, rather than providing for others, she is the one being cared for. The father who is ill may experience similar dynamics, now no longer the repository of strength, now unable to secure the family's well-being by word and deed. Illness creates upheaval in the family system. Children become parents to their parents, and parents feel reduced to the dependency of children. Husbands and wives become afraid of intimacy, as they need to adapt to the other's condition and redefine the parameters of their relationship. The effect of illness on families is to make members unsure of their place and role. Communication suffers as each becomes a familiar stranger to their kin.

The manifestation of this estrangement is often subtle. A woman described her relationship to her husband, hospitalized with cancer. Early on when she said good-bye she kissed him. As the illness progressed and her husband became more the patient and less the lover, she ran her hand over his cheek when saying good-bye. Later, she noted, to say good-bye meant touching his feet at the end of the bed. By the end, good-bye was simply a wave. The sick and, yes, their families are not unaffected by the diminished intimacy. The change in engagement patterns is slow and often hidden to the eye. But over time the sick and their families disconnect. The banter and spontaneous conversation is frequently lost. In the anxiety over the inability to articulate with each other their fears and frustrations, family members avoid the sick, or are silent in their presence, or worse yet become busy bees of activity over-involved in attending to the needs of the patient, hoping no one will recognize the truth of their inability to communicate.

Caregivers frequently make a seriously erroneous assumption as they enter the world of the sick and their families. They assume that in illness, family members are drawn closer together. After all they see the ever-present wife or child at the bedside. The caregivers expect the challenge to the family survival now present to engender a solidarity of purpose expressed in greater intimacy. The caregivers imagine that all the tensions of relationships will dissolve in this moment of crisis. The caregivers will often project this love on to the scene. They will affirm the devotion, closeness, intimacy, regardless of its truth.

More likely the opposite is true.

When Jacob sustains the loss of Joseph, he becomes distant from his family. Yes, they all rise up to comfort him. Superficially they are present to each other. But Jacob refuses to be comforted and remains alone.

When Isaac and Rebecca are pained over their inability to conceive, the Torah tells us that they prayed "opposite" each other.[11] In tradition, each went to different corners. The stress and disappointment produced not greater intimacy, but more isolation. Childlessness was a problem they shared. But because of their differences of person and role, it was experienced privately. There was no "we," only "I" as they struggled to come to terms with their unique story of loss.

Crisis stresses families. It challenges communication patterns. Most often it causes, over time, family members to feel more alienated as the personal experience of their situations go unexpressed.

It is this otherness in one's predicament in the context of the family he/she loves that heightens the experience of suffering. Typically, each family member wants to protect the other, pretend it will be all right, even though all too often even in the best of circumstances nothing will ever be the same. Afraid to face the sadness in the other should the truth be known, afraid to acknowledge the reality of roles now turned on their heads, family members engage in games and well-intentioned lies. The result of this well-meaning dance of pretence is to cause deeper and more painful isolation. Secretly the family engages in an unspoken collusion in which each member in his/her heart knows the truth, but all conspire to "act as if" it were otherwise.

At the deepest level of estrangement, illness alienates a person from him/herself. Sick, unable, despondent, afraid the person loses his/her core sense of identity. The person looks in the mirror and does not recognize him/herself. Illness has robbed the person of his/her form. He/she struggles to accept the broken condition of his/her body. It seems so contrary to the self-image he/she carried for so long. The person used to lift weights, and now cannot even lift his/her arm. The person once controlled a company and now cannot control his/her own bowel movements. The sick, in the beginning, think it a bad dream from which they will soon awake, a dream in which some variant form has claimed their person and body. Gradually over time they forget the "they" that was the

---

11. Genesis 25:21

dreamer and get lost in the dream. They no longer even remember the other healthy self prior to the onset of their problem. In losing their self, they lose their personal power. They become mute, silent, numb to their own circumstances. Gone is the "I" of the experience. They have become their illness.

This is the deepest and most painful kind of suffering, the suffering of losing one's self. To the world outside the person may appear compliant, quiet, even accepting of his/her situation. In truth the person is so disconnected from his/her experience that he/she is already "dead" to him/herself and the world. The isolation is so painful that it numbs him/her into acquiescence. He/she no longer feels. Even to say "I want" feels impossible. Is it any surprise then in medical institutions, when patients are already so disconnected from themselves, that filling out healthcare proxies would be near impossible? Persons reduced to patients have a hard time filling out a menu, never mind making decisions on end-of-life treatment plans. The symptoms often manifest themselves as depression. In truth, it is much worse. The person has checked out. What's left is an empty form, a pale image of the original.

Ginny was a case in point. I met her when she was in her early fifties. She came as a student to Clinical Pastoral Education (CPE). Ginny was a Roman Catholic nun, good-hearted with a sweetness born of innocence. What I noted about Ginny was how her speech seemed clipped, almost childlike. She rarely spoke more than a sentence or two at a time, and even then it was usually in response to my or another's query. When she spoke she was painfully deliberate, as if each word was a struggle to verbalize. Over time I came to know Ginny and learned her story. She had been seriously abused as a child. At times, she was so neglected as to be left at home, tied up, as her parents left the house for hours. Alone, helpless, with no one to hear her cries, she became mute, unable to speak. Her suffering turned her inward to such a degree that she lost all ability to have intercourse with the world without. She lost her self. Only years later through a painstaking treatment process did Ginny learn to communicate. First she simply learned to mumble, to make guttural sounds to express feelings. Later she gained access to verbal self-expression. By the time I met her she would pass for "normal" if different. But in truth even as a woman in her fifties every effort to bring her feelings out into the world of expression was a challenge.

While rarely do the sick suffer the loss of self to the extent of Ginny's experience, it is not uncommon to note the silence of those suffering prolonged illness. At times that quiet is attributed to depression. In spiritual language we call it despair. What we may not realize is that the silence often reflects not the lost voice, but rather the lost person as the *Galut* of the illness experience has reached its deepest level. Healing then becomes the work of the resurrection of the dead.

Chapter 3
The Gift of Healing Relationship

> *Rabbi Hiya, son of Abba became ill.*
>
> *Rabbi Yochanan went to visit him. He said to him, "Do you like these afflictions?"*
>
> *"I like neither them nor their reward," Rabbi Hiya replied.*
>
> *Rabbi Yochanan then invited Rabbi Hiya to give him his hand. Rabbi Hiya gave his hand to Rabbi Yochanan and he healed him.*[1]

This Talmudic story tells us much about the work of healing. Healing requires a relationship. No matter how much Rabbi Yochanan may want for Rabbi Hiya to recover, unless Rabbi Hiya can affirm his own desire to get well, Rabbi Yochanan will be powerless to heal him. It is not clear what the nature of Rabbi Hiya's illness was. The Talmud, in truth, does not say, "Rabbi Yochanan cured Rabbi Hiya." Nor does it say, "He healed him." Rather it says, "He got him up." The implication here is that we are dealing with circumstances in which suffering may be the operative issue. We may speculate that the actual disease affecting Rabbi Hiya had passed. Yet he languished. It was for that very reason that Rabbi Yochanan challenged him to ascertain his commitment to recovery and bolster his resolve.

This understanding of the dynamics becomes more likely when we read the following story in the Talmud. This time Rabbi

---

1. Brachot 5b

Yochanan himself was ill. He was visited by Rabbi Channinah. Rabbi Channinah challenged Rabbi Yochanan's resolve to get well in the same way Rabbi Yochanan challenged Rabbi Hiya earlier. Then, once assured of Rabbi Yochanan's desire to recover, Rabbi Channinah and Rabbi Yochanan hold hands and he is "lifted up" out of his illness. The Talmud then asks the obvious question. Since Rabbi Yochanan was clearly knowing of the healing arts, why did he need Rabbi Channinah to heal him? He should have been able to heal himself. It answers, "A prisoner cannot free himself from his own jail cell."[2]

What is the meaning of the metaphor as it relates to our story? True, a prisoner cannot release himself from jail. The lock is on the outside of the door! How does the prisoner metaphor explain Rabbi Yochanan's powerlessness to self-heal? Moreover, if we were focused on cure why can't an individual who is him/herself a physician prescribe the necessary medication or treatment and get well? And if a physician cannot successfully diagnose and medicate him/herself, why is it necessary to make reference to a prisoner? What does the metaphor add?

The answer is that our story's theme is not about the practice of medicine. Rather it is about healing and restoring a person to a sense of wellness. Even if a person is cured of the physical circumstances that compromise him/her, he/she still needs to reclaim his/her self. The residue of illness is the impact of the experience of suffering. As we discussed in the prior chapter, suffering causes estrangement. It alienates a person from core components of his/her identity. It leaves an individual disconnected from the energy that motivates him/her and that animates his/her existence. Rabbi Yochanan saw Rabbi Hiya and knew that what he needed was self-renewal, release from the consequences of suffering. When Rabbi Yochanan became ill, indeed he could take care of his own physical impairment. But our story is about suffering. The suffering are like the prisoners, who in their incarceration have lost themselves and no matter the change of external circumstances cannot reclaim life in freedom without the help of others. Yes, they may

2. Brachot 5b

no longer be constrained. But they still see themselves as trapped and disempowered. As in the story of imprisonment, healing is in a profound way about liberation, liberation of the eclipsed and alienated self. Liberation requires both the resolve of the person and the assistance of another who helps that person find that part of his/her inner identity that has always lived beyond incarceration and remained forever free.

Caregiving is a response to suffering. The one core element of the work is building a healing relationship with those experiencing suffering. For it is only through aligning ourselves with the alienated and estranged suffering that they can begin the process of self-renewal necessary to reclaim wellness. Support groups that have become commonplace for every sort of person in recovery from cancer survivors to incest survivors give evidence to the veracities of suffering's lingering impact and that the way to healing inevitably requires relationships of alignment. Without the support of caring others ready to meet the suffering in their state of exile, it may be impossible for them to ever become whole again. Yes they may be disease-free or passed the trauma, but they will remain in some significant way disconnected from their true selves and spiritually compromised. A part of them will be mute even as Ginny was mute, and while we may not define it as suffering, there is no greater tragedy than the acceptance of a destiny not one's own, no greater suffering than one so profound as to no longer be voiced or raised to consciousness.

It is important for us here to make the distinction between healing and cure. Practitioners of the medical sciences are engaged in curing. Chaplains, rabbis, and those providing social services are primarily invested in healing. Curing is focused on disease. Healing focuses on the person. Curing is about treatment. Healing concerns itself with relationship. The works are not only different, in some important ways they are mutually exclusive. Let us explore the idea of healing from its source. The Talmud derives the *mitzvot* of doing *hesed* from our responsibility to follow in God's way. Just as God visited the sick, so must we. Just as God comforted the mourners, so must we. Just as God clothed the naked, so must we.[3] *Bikur cholim* and *nichum aveilim* are the specific areas of caregiving of which we are concerned inasmuch as they are *mitzvot* that require extension of oneself in the expression of care to be fulfilled.

The Talmud goes on to discuss *bikur cholim* and to identify God's visit to our father Abraham in the beginning of the portion of *Vayaira* as an instance of God visiting the sick. They point out, Abraham was then recovering from his circumcision, discussed in the earlier verses. God's visit to Abraham becomes then the paradigm for us who are then called upon to follow in God's ways.[4] Yet, we might ask, how does the Talmud know that visitation of the sick was the reason for God's appearance to Abraham? There is no mention in the Torah verses of the topic discussed or the reason for God's revealed presence. All the verse says is "And God appeared to him in the terebinths of Mamreh…"[5] The answer is that we know *bikur cholim* was God's intent because God's appearance is never followed with an explanation as to the reason for the appearance. There is no commandment, prophetic vision, or tiding here. All the Torah tells us is that "God appeared." Clearly, then, the visit was not the means to achieve some external end. The visit is the end. God's purpose was simply to be with Abraham. This becomes even more apparent when we examine the structure of the verse. Literally, the verse translates "And appeared to him God…," the object preceding the subject of the sentence, highly irregular in Torah usage. More typically, we would have expected it to read "And God appeared to Abraham…" In the structure of the verse, we get confirmation that "to him" is the crucial locus of the activity and its *raison d'être*. Even God subordinates God's self to make Abraham, not God, the center of the experience. That all makes sense if God's purpose was *bikur cholim*, where relationship is the central dimension of the *mitzvah*, and the focus of the visit needs to be about the person ill, not the visitor, even if the visitor is God.

---

3. BT Sota 14a

4. Ibid

5. Genesis 18:1

Clearly then the Torah passage telling us about God's kindness of visiting the sick is revealing not only of the fact that this is the way of the Divine and we, under the imperative *imitatio Dei*, are expected to do likewise. The Torah passage provides us with the way the *mitzvah* is to be done, the context of the *mitzvah*. We are taught here not only the "what" of this *hesed* but the "how." God's appearance is designed to foster relationship with Abraham. To do so, God needs to let Abraham decide on the mood, the content and the theme of their time together. *Bikur cholim* is never about what the visitor brings into the room of the sick, some wise Torah teaching, some inspiring story, some humorous anecdote. No, on the contrary, what goes on in the visit must emerge from the sick person, his/her need and mindset. The role of the visitor is to let go of the stuff he/she has on his/her plate so as to be as God was with Abraham, totally free to meet the sick other in an I-Thou encounter.

The remainder of this episode in early Genesis provides even more guidance to the work of healing *hesed*. Abraham saw three strangers on the road. He rushed out to meet them in order to provide them hospitality. The Talmud teaches us that they were in fact three angels with three different responsibilities, one of them assigned to cure Abraham.[6] Now that is quite surprising. Why did God need to send an angel to cure Abraham? God was already visiting him. What was the difference between God's visit and the angel's mission? Why could not God both visit and cure? Here the Torah makes clear to us that *bikur cholim* is about healing, not cure. When God visited Abraham, if God would have cured him, Abraham would have been free of pain, but he would still have the lingering sense of limitation caused by suffering. The angel treated Abraham's wound. God affirmed Abraham as a person, honoring him as whole even in his state of physical pain and diminishment. Those engaged in curative efforts cannot be instruments of healing. Their very focus on the disease, and symptoms, puts them in the one-up position and affirms the sick as being in need of fixing and help. Caregiving as expressed in the work of *bikur cholim* and

6. BT Bava Metziah p86b

nichum aveilim is an effort in healing. It requires the cultivation of relationship. While curing may be designated to angels, healing belongs to God.

So now that we have established that the work of caregiving requires the development of a healing relationship, we need to explore the dynamics of this relationship and how it is achieved. The Talmud tells us "Any one who visits the sick removes one sixtieth of their suffering".[7] It then immediately qualifies the statement by saying "This is only true however if the visitor is a *ben gilo*. *Ben gilo* is an interesting term. It has been translated in some commentaries as being in the same age group as the one who is ill.[8] Others translate the meaning of *ben gil* as being born under the same astrological sign as the one ill.[9] Clearly the implication is that to remove suffering one needs to align oneself with the sick in the most profound way. While other visitors may relieve some of the implications of suffering, only the *ben gil*, one who understands the experience of the other at the deepest level, either because he/she has a similar temperament (symbolized in being born under the same sign) or is of similar age can achieve the full impact of reducing the sufferer's distress by one sixtieth. To establish a healing relationship, the caregiver needs to become as much as possible a *ben gil* to the sick and suffering. He/she needs to find within him/herself a point of connection with the other at the place the other inhabits. While the occasional visitor may naturally be a *ben gil*, the professional caregiver, chaplain, rabbi, social worker, he/she must find the aspect of their own story, personality, makeup that will match the experience of the other so as to build a community of the alone.

Where do we find this component of ourselves? How can we simply be expected to dial-up a *ben gil* within? What number can we use? Henri Nouwen in his classic work in the field of pastoral care, *The Wounded Healer*, argues that all clergy have a dimension of woundedness within (and by association we might argue all

---

7. Nedarim 39b

8. Rashi, Nedarim 39b

9. Ibid

caregivers). To build a community with the sick and suffering, the clergy must access their own sense of woundedness and establish an alignment with the wounded other.[10] What is called for is not the clergyperson's excellence, or virtue. He/she is not meant to represent perfection. Rather it is the clergyperson's woundedness that must match the woundedness of the other and build a bridge to span the chasm between the world of the healthy and the world of the sick. Nouwen, drawing on his Christian tradition, charges the caregivers to imitate Jesus, who, in his understanding, accessed his woundedness as the point of connection to heal others.[11] We have no tradition of a wounded messiah, or of any imperative to emulate the messiah in ourselves. On the contrary, we are charged to imitate God's ways, not God's being. Where, we might question, is our point of reference? The wounded healer might be a paradigm that works for Christians. It does not however match Jewish experience or Jewish theology.

In truth, Judaism has its own paradigm for the healing relationship. The image caregivers are called to actualize has its roots deep in our national consciousness. It is core to both our experience and our identity. The Torah makes it clear. "And you shall love the stranger".[12] Forty-five times the Torah calls upon us in one form or another to be sensitive to the marginalization of the outsider. No, even more, the Torah demands of us to love the stranger. Yet, we might well ask, keep the Sabbath and it can be done; give *Tzedekah* (charity), and we know what our mandate is. The *mitzvot* are challenges to behavior. They are practices we can perform, albeit, at times, with difficulty. But ask of us to "love the stranger," and we might well wonder how. How can we cause in ourselves a feeling if not truly present? We can make ourselves eat, but we are never commanded to be hungry. Love is likewise a feeling, beyond the ability to will or demand of ourselves. How can the Torah expect it of us? Moreover, how can we engender in ourselves the love the

10. Henri J.M. Nouwen, *The Wounded Healer* (Garden City, NY; Image Books, 1979) pp 82ff

11. Ibid p 94

12. Deuteronomy 10:19

Torah calls for?

The answer lies in the words that follow. "And you shall love the stranger" in the Torah narrative. It reads "for you were strangers in the land of Egypt".[13] We can love the stranger because we know the experience of being a stranger. We have within us the aware- ness of the suffering attendant to being on the outside trying to find acceptance of community. We have embedded within our psyche the suffering that is born out of our encounter in Egypt, in which we were the oppressed marginalized. We can love the stranger, in- deed we must love the stranger, because he/she is living a story that is ours as well. In finding the "stranger" in ourselves, we will feel a natural empathy with every stranger, an empathy that is rooted in love. To love the stranger all we need to do is align ourselves with our own national story, know who we are as a people. To love the other will then be no more difficult than loving ourselves.

The paradigm for providing care emerging from our tradition is not the "wounded healer" of Nouwen. It is the image of the "stranger," so central to our identity as Jews that impels us. For as we have discussed, the suffering of the sick and for that matter all suffering has its roots in a sense of estrangement. In entering the world of the suffering, our challenge is to find that "stranger" experience we know so well and call it up, so that we may live in it, if only for a while, and become the *ben gil* for the estranged other. We need to summon from out collective unconscious our story of living life disconnected and alone, the experience of Egypt we are challenged over and over to remember. In taking on the place of the estranged in society, we are enabled in ways that are surprising. Ironically, in becoming aligned with our own sense of otherness, we can build an alignment with the alone other, ill and suffering, and realize a healing that was unavailable for us to achieve in our complacency and normal state of belonging.

In its broadest sense, the caregiving relationship can be accom- plished as our "stranger" meets the stranger in the bed and creates a community of the alone. We become a *ben gil* in our common story of estrangement. At a deeper level, our challenge is to find

13. Deuteronomy 10:19

in ourselves a more particular identification with the specific story of the person we are visiting that the other may know a *ben gil* not only in the general terms of their suffering story but even in its individual expression. When a patient's estrangement shows up as fear of an impending surgery and its consequences, we must listen well to what exactly the other is afraid of. We need to draw out from him/her the content of his/her worry. We must not assume we know the source of the fear or its quality. One person may be afraid of dying, another afraid of living. Even one afraid of dying may fear perhaps the pain of death or perhaps the experience of leaving behind one's loved ones or perhaps something else entirely. We cannot know the truth of the other's suffering unless and until we engage him/her with an open ear and a curious heart. To become a *ben gil*, establish a relationship that repairs the suffering rooted in a deep sense of aloneness and estrangement, we need to invest ourselves in discerning the story of the suffering in the context of his/her life. Making a quick diagnosis of the feeling of the person we are visiting and then assuming we know him/her and his/her story may only cause the sick a deeper sense of emotional isolation, for here we seemed to invite a healing intimacy only to then impose our experience on him/her. The sick may accept our interpretations out of a lack of energy or even faith in their own truth. They may not ever tell us how wrong we were about the truth of their inner struggle. We may leave the room certain we connected and established a healing I-Thou encounter with the sick. And yet because we failed to listen adequately we only pushed the sick deeper into their experience of estrangement as they acquiesced as another person, perhaps even a rabbi, told them who they are and what they should be experiencing.

To become a *ben gil* first and foremost we must learn to listen to the person we are visiting. Listening takes time. If we do not have time we had better simply acknowledge our limitation and not pretend to offer the depth of care we cannot offer authentically. In listening we need be attentive not only to the illness story but to the story of the other's hopes, dreams, disappointments and expectations. We need to know what meaning he/she attaches to his/her illness, how the story does or does not fit for him/her in the larger script of his/her life. In inviting the other to share his/her story, we are inviting the suffering to rediscover the self he/she has become estranged from. We are beginning the process of healing, in which the sick can be whole even in times of disease and distress.

Listening to the other is more than a work of the mind. We are not listening to gain knowledge as if we were studying some exotic species. We are listening with our heart in order to draw near. We listen as a way to understand, so that we can achieve the intimacy born of a sense of communion. We do not listen by posing questions. Questions engender an imbalance in relationship. The one asking questions has power, the one answering is surrendering control, hardly a model for alignment of equals. Rather we share conversation with the suffering other. We listen and follow and let the other be revealed, not as a series of facts collected, but as a person unfolding before us, in his/her own time, in his/her own way. As we listen, we seek to find in ourselves places of identification with the other. We do not always, or even often, share our place of identification, but nonetheless we are thereby engaged so that we can let the other know by our manner, mood and expression that we are with him/her, that we are coming to understand him/her and value him/her and the power of his/her story. And so we as *ben gil* effect a parallel process. As the sick and suffering find an alignment with us, as patients, engaged with aligned listeners, they also connect to their own truer selves. In telling the story they have lost and now rediscover, they reclaim the self they were before they surrendered their identities as persons in order to become patients. They attain a renewed sense of wholeness and hope.

Engendering the reclamation of self that relieves suffering is not a one-step process. As in the story of Ginny referenced earlier, the suffering need encouragement to find their voices. Often through the weeks, months and at times years of estrangement and self-diminishment, the suffering lose connection to their story, as well as their personhood. Only through patient attentiveness will the suffering be able to give voice to their deeper truths and once again know the life force lost. The caregiver must realize that even if he/she knows what the suffering will say, knows their story and experience, perhaps due to prior history with them or even due to its having been shared in a prior visit, it nonetheless may be of great importance for the suffering to speak it. The very process of articulation is restorative. In telling their story, the suffering are reclaiming their personal power. Each time told it unblocks a clogged passageway to the lost self.

Early in my own experience in Clinical Pastoral Education, I visited a non-Jewish patient on one of my assigned units. We had a deep conversation concerning his doubts over his future and his regret for past misdeeds. As I was leaving, the pastor of his church, with whom he had a long-term relationship, stopped by for a visit. The pastor later complained that his parishioner seemed more engaged with me than with him. What the pastor did not understand was that at times familiarity is unhelpful in cultivating a healing relationship.

Knowing a person well may cause us to frame his/her story for him/her. He/she may have little room to share his/her experience in a new way, cast his/her life in a context different from the commonly accepted one. The suffering benefit at times from being cared for by someone wholly unfamiliar with their past. It allows them to speak the fullness of their heart and be known as they want to be, rather than as publicly perceived.

Typically, Jewish students in Clinical Pastoral Education will express great surprise at the openness with which those of other faiths and even other ethnic/racial backgrounds share deep concerns with them. What is even more surprising is how often Jewish patients share more deeply with non-Jewish chaplains than with rabbis, their own or the community's.

Let me share here a verbatim account of a visit between an African-American Muslim chaplain-intern and a Jewish patient that illustrates both the unique rapport achieved across religious and racial differences, and the reasons why.

Muhammad was a 30-year-old chaplain-intern at Beth Israel Medical Center. He was an African-American Muslim participating in CPE. In the encounter described below, he visited with

Nachman, a 32-year-old Modern-Orthodox Jew, on one of his assigned units. His goal was to provide spiritual support while respectful of a person's unique beliefs and practices.

C1: Hi. My name is Muhammad. I am the chaplain here on this unit.
P1: Hi. My name is Nachman. Are you a Muslim?

C2: Yes.
P2: Salam.

C3: Shalom. How are you doing?
P3: Better. I am stuck here.

C4: What brought you here?
P4: I have pneumonia. The doctors say I need to take the medications and clear my lungs.

C5: That sounds frightening.
P5: You think so?

C6: Well for me it would be!
P6: I am surprised. I didn't think a Muslim would say that.

C7: How come?
P7: Because you take life as a test like we Jews do. You are supposed to have faith.

C8: That's true. But hey that doesn't mean I wouldn't be frightened or scared.
P8: Hmm. Never thought of it that way.

C9: So how do you see it?
P9: Well according to the Torah, God gives and takes away life as He sees fit. So, in this moment, God is testing me.

C10: Now, see, that scares me!
P10: It does?

C11: Sure it does. I don't even know when God will call me back.
P11: That's interesting. I never express that outside myself. But inside I was wrestling with my own fears.

Muhammad and Nachman then went on to have an intimate conversation in which Nachman shared some of the difficulties he had holding to the Orthodoxy of his youth and his recent return to the way of observance. In the end Nachman asked Muhammad to return the next day. Each bid the other farewell in the language of their tradition.

At once the visit is surprising and revealing. Nachman and Muhammad are of different ethnic backgrounds, racially different, and of different religions. Yet in a graceful way they connect. The bridge between them is their shared sense of being strangers in a society not their own. Each is in some important way alone. They are of the same *gil* in terms of age. More profoundly, they are of the same *gil* in terms of feeling marginalized. In that common sense of being outsiders, they forge community. Nachman was able to claim his self in terms of both feeling and story. It was a poignant "healing" moment.

In essence, the challenge posed to caregivers is really two-fold. At one level they need to resist their own anxiety around the suffering so they can be available to be present without distancing themselves through "helping" or "fixing," as we discussed in the opening chapter. In order to attain that comfort level, they need at once to both identify with the person and their predicament and yet recognize at a deep level that the story of the suffering is not their own. They need to have clear boundaries in discerning whose problem this is and whose it is not. And yet paradoxically, at the very same time that the caregivers need to establish boundaries that engender distance, they also need to build intimacy by joining with the suffering in the predicament of suffering. They need to look into themselves and their stories so as to find the ground of meeting and become a *ben gil*. The caregiver needs to access his/her own experience and life journey to help build community with the other. Yet at the same time he/she needs to be forever mindful that the story here is not his/her story. Rather it is the story of the one being cared for.

Caregiving challenges us to a dance of intimacy, one in which respect for the otherness of the one receiving care is balanced by our love born out of nearness. It is forever an imperfect act. At times we may find the sufferer too difficult to respect as other. We cannot embrace him/her for we cannot tolerate either who he/she is or what he/she is coping with. Ultimately, that inability to embrace is born out of fear, fear that nearness to the other as either person or sufferer will affect us.

We struggle to recognize sufficiently the uniqueness and inherent otherness of the person for whom we are caring. At times, we find love for the other impossible to attain. His/her situation feels so foreign to us, so other, that we remain detached emotionally, clinically present but absent of personal investment. Most of the time we wrestle with ourselves on the continuum between what some would call over identifying with the suffering and on the other pole being unaffected. In our work as caregivers, we need to consistently question ourselves in relationship with the suffering other so as to be available to the optimum in intimacy.

Instances where nearness may make us too anxious to be present with respect for the unique experience of the sufferer often occurs when we have had similar experiences and have not fully processed them. The chaplain who is visiting a similar age woman soon to have a mastectomy and who has not fully grieved her own breast cancer experience may indeed be too close to care without being overwhelmed. The rabbi who was abused by authority in his own childhood experience may feel compelled to offer advice when the child of a congregant complains of mistreatment at home. The rabbi's own repression of his/her experience may make it impossible for him/her to hear the other's story without reactivity. In most cases, our urge to run away by fixing, helping or minimizing is rooted in connections to the other of which we are unaware. The over-identification has its source in personal material lodged in our unconscious, not only unprocessed but unknown to us. Not surprisingly, then, to become effective as a caregiver we need to know ourselves and our story. We must come to explore fully what we bring into relationship with another so that we will be free to meet the other without impediments caused by material in our own lives we are too afraid to confront. Clinical Pastoral Education is an appropriate requisite for certification as a spiritual caregiver inasmuch as the education process challenges students to come to terms with their own autobiographical material even as it teaches pastoral skills. To the extent that we are unaware of the reactivity triggered in us by those we are called to help, we risk not only failing to help them, but actually in our unconsciousness, we may further their experience of isolation and diminishment. In our self-ignorance we may well do harm in the guise of caring.

Our tendency to see the sufferer as too other from us to emotionally attach represents for us a different challenge. Perhaps the one cared for is so much older than we are as to be beyond our place of identification or too different in cultural/religious background, gender or life circumstance. In all these circumstances, to engender a healing relationship and become a *ben gil*, we need to listen carefully to the story of the other so that we might find points that stir our emotions. Even as the other tells his/her story, we need to be open to our own experience to access life moments that will bridge the divide.

As we discussed earlier, we are all "strangers" and at least at that level can join the hurting other. In more subtle ways, the unique struggle of each person can be found in some dimensions of all of our experience. We all have known grief, loss, shame, guilt, despair, anger, even if the individual stories are different in urgency, depth, and detail. In listening with our hearts, we can find the shared and, while respectful of the other's experience, join him/her in it.

Excellence in caregiving here requires us to have access to a wide repertoire of diverse and multi-layered experiences within, so that we can become a *ben gil* to as wide a group of persons as we may meet. Here, too, as in the challenge to not be too near, the call to find the common impels us to self-exploration. We must be available to all of ourselves, even that of which we feel less than pleased, so that we can summon it up to establish places in common with the suffering other who evidences feelings and attitudes we might disdain.

Often I hear the comment from caregivers "…all I really did was listen" as if listening itself is the central work of facilitating healing. While in truth listening is a most important focus of the activity of *hesed*, as we have described it, and it certainly avoids the traps of "fixing" and "helping," it is not enough. To do the work of *hesed*, in keeping with the challenge of its source "love thy neighbor as thyself," we need to do more than listen. We need to resonate with the other's experience so as to become companions with him/her on his/her journey, mitigating the aloneness and engendering a restorative alignment that returns the person to him/herself.

It is important here to note that the self that we as caregivers invite the sufferer to reclaim may not be the old self that he/she lived out of prior to his/her illness story. On the contrary, Judaism has long seen life as a teacher and all that happens to us as opportunities Divinely granted that we might achieve a wholeness or *shlaimut* we have not yet realized.

While none of us can say what the reason for our life's circumstances may be, tradition tells us that the experiences of our lives are purposive and by design. What occurs to us is meant for us to live as fully as possible and grow from. In cultivating a healing relationship, we help the suffering other to enter their story of suffering rather than run away from it. We accompany the other so as to give him/her the strength and courage to draw from the experience what might be important for his/her development. The self we help the other rediscover may be one that even the other had as yet not fully known. The caregiver, by entering into a healing relationship with the other in the deepest sense, becomes a conduit to help the sufferer make meaning out of his/her experience and become whole in a new way. The caregiver does more than sustain and revive. In building a healing relationship, the caregiver is the instrument of hope and reformation. We will explore the unique and sacred dimension to the work of caregiving in the next chapter.

Chapter 4
The Rabbi as Pastor

Rabbi Shimon bar Yochai, the Talmudic sage and mystic, once went to perform the mitzvah of bikur cholim. He met a man with his stomach distended suffering with an intestinal disease who, in his misery, was cursing the Divine over his circumstances.

Rabbi Shimon said to him, "Empty one, you should be praying for mercy, and instead, you utter obscenities to God!"

The man replied, "God should take the suffering from me and put it on you!"

Reflecting on the encounter, Rabbi Shimon ben Yochai observed, "I got what I deserved from the Holy One Blessed Be He, for I forsook the words of Torah for idle chatter."[1]

The above, excerpted from the Talmudic text Avot of Rabbi Nathan, is surprising in many ways. Rabbi Shimon bar Yochai according to tradition was the greatest of mystics. He is reported to be the author of the Zohar, the source text for the Kabbalah. He, above all his great colleagues, penetrated the secrets of the world and its creation. How could he fail so miserably to be sensitive to the dynamics of his fellow human being? Moreover, if indeed he hoped to move this suffering man to a renewed love of God despite his awful illness, his method evidenced so little understanding of people and their temperaments.

1. Avot D'Rabbi Natan 41:1

Rabbi Shimon bar Yochai not only failed to do the *hesed* he set out for, he in fact made this man's situation worse. The great rabbi insulted him, called him "empty one!"

And the above story is not the only one of its kind. The Talmud in another place tells the story of Rabbi Yochanan ben Zakai, who sustained the tragic death of his son. Five of his great students, all rabbis of note themselves and all men of wisdom and character, came to comfort him, one at a time. First Rabbi Eliezer sat with his Rebbe. He tried to comfort Rabbi Yochanan by comparing his loss to Adam's, who sustained the death of his son Abel and nonetheless renewed his commitment to life. Rabbi Yochanan responded, "Is it not enough I have my own suffering to endure – you want to remind me of the suffering of Adam."[2] In succession, Rabbi Joshua, Rabbi Josie and Rabbi Shimon visited their Rebbe Rabbi Yochanan. Each in turn attempted to bring comfort by comparing Rabbi Yochanan's loss to an earlier father whose son(s) had died, in one case Job, in another Aaron, in a third David. In each case, Rabbi Yochanan responded as he did to Rabbi Eliezer, saying essentially "you only made my suffering worse by adding to my loss the loss of another." Only Rabbi Elazar ben Arach, the last of the five students/rabbis, brought a measure of comfort in affirming that Rabbi Yochanan had done a good job as father to his wonderful son even as he need endure the inconsolable pain of his son's death.

Here, too, we are surprised at how rabbis of historic greatness fail so miserably at the *mitzvah* of *nichum aveilim*, comforting the mourners. How is it that men so versed in Torah and so rich in personal integrity and character could so miss the moment and offer words that not only compromised their intent, but words that in fact engendered more suffering and exacerbated the sense of loss?

What becomes clear on reflection is that the work of caregiving requires a personal development of self not only not available through Torah study but in many ways in stark contrast to it. The study of Torah challenges the Jew to access the enduring, spiritual, uncompromising part of his/herself. Truth and the pursuit of truth is the object. Emotions, ego needs, personality, only get in the

---

2. Avot D'Rabbi Natan 14:6

way. Objectivity is what is called for. One needs to transcend one's earthly limitations to maximize the experience. In Malachi we read, "For priests' lips should preserve knowledge and they should seek the law at his mouth, for he is a messenger of the Lord of hosts."[3] The sages of the Talmud understood the text to say, "Only if the teacher is comparable to an angel of the Lord of hosts should you study Torah from him."[4] To be excellent in Torah and appropriate in transmitting Torah to others, one needs to cultivate the perfection and other-worldliness of an angel. It is not surprising that the rabbis in the stories above would fail to empathize with their grieving teacher in one case and with the suffering man in the other. Angels have no way to feel the feelings of another. They cannot become a *ben gil*. When God visited Abraham in the Torah story from which we learn the *mitzvah* of *bikur cholim*, God sends three angels disguised as men. One of them was sent specifically to cure Abraham as he was recovering from his wound (in tradition the result of his circumcision). It is worth noting that God visited while the angel cured. On reflection, who might wonder why cure did not become the prerogative of the Divine, since it seems a more significant act. Why didn't God cure and let the angel visit? The answer is that angels by definition cannot visit if visiting means engendering intimacy with a human. Angels can cure, angels can wrestle (the story of Jacob), angels can instruct (the encounter with Balaam). To the extent that one has succeeded in one's Torah study and becomes as an angel, one will be unavailable to the work *hesed* requires of identification with the suffering other. The more in fact one excels in Torah, the more difficult it will be to cultivate healing relationships.

In order to become a resource for healing, rabbis and others need to gain access to their earthy selves, the part of them that gets angry, resentful, selfish, afraid and cynical. The caregiver has to dial into his/her inner channel to locate the frequency that will allow him/her to meet the wounded and suffering where they are. Rabbi Shimon bar Yochai could not likely find any bitterness

---

3. Malachi 2:7

4. Hagigah 15b

toward God in himself, even with all the struggles of his own life. He was indeed a *Tzadik*. But he was not the right person to visit the bitter and angry man with intestinal disease. To successfully be a source of comfort and restoration in that context only a rabbi or other who could resonate with the feelings of resentment, even toward God, could become a healing presence.

In light of the above, it should not be surprising to find that many rabbis and seminary students with all their Jewish learning are poorly equipped for the work of relationship building in the challenge of providing care. The world they come from is a world of Torah study. Their ideal is the pursuit of truth. In caregiving the objective truth does not matter near as much as the personal truth experienced by the suffering. The congregational rabbi who may be an exemplar in modeling Jewish devotion and piety is often deficient in empathy. He/she may be wonderful at mobilizing resources to help the poor. He/she may be a forceful advocate for change. He/she may have the zeal of a prophet to rail against society's human evils. But at the bedside or in the intimate office encounter, he/she will often not know how to become a companion to the wounded in their story and state. When seminary students enroll in Clinical Pastoral Education much of the work is remedial. The person on the street may have more capacity to feel with the sick and alone than the budding rabbi. After all, the person on the street lives with his/her mediocrity and earthy limitations. The seminarian has spent years in both formal and informal settings striving to rise above his/her limitations in identifying with the Godly.

In describing the way of Torah, the Mishna teaches, "This is the way of Torah: Eat bread with salt, drink water in small measure, sleep on the ground, live a life of deprivation, but toil in the Torah!…"[5] Compare that with what Avot of Rabbi Nathan tells us at the conclusion of the story of the students or Rabbi Yochanan ben Zakai. All the four who failed to bring comfort to their Rebbe, we are told, went on to settle in Yavneh, a place of great scholarship and devotion to Torah study. Rabbi Elazar ben Arach, on the

---

5. Avot 6:4

other hand, decided to settle in Damasis, a place of geographical beauty and excellent water. The passage goes on to say that the four students, consistent with their choice, became more prominent in Torah, while Rabbi Elazar ben Arach, consistent with his choice, had his reputation in Torah diminished as a consequence.[6]

The implications of the story are clear. While the four rabbis failed miserably to bring comfort, they pursued the way of Torah study and teaching. Rabbi Elazar ben Arach, in bringing comfort, had to access his earthy side, the part of himself that enjoyed life's pleasures and lived with the blessings and curses of finitude. The way of the one who brings healing relationship is one of immersion in the world. The way of Torah is the way of detachment. Each has its brilliance. Each has its cost. While rabbis and seminarians are dedicated to Torah, if they aspire to serve in a congregational context and provide *hesed* in an exemplary manner they will need to balance the devotion to the Torah with its attendant detachment from the material, with a relationship with life and its inherent compromises, so as to be able to identify with the suffering and become for them a *ben gil*.

While one might expect the need to develop one's earthy self is more an issue with Orthodox rabbis and seminarians, my experience as a pastoral educator has shown me that the need for remediation is as much a need for those identifying with the other streams of Judaism. Let me share an incident illustrative of the problem. I attended the wedding of a middle-aged couple, each getting married for the second time. Both had children from their previous marriages and they decided on a home wedding where those children would be in attendance. They each chose a rabbi who knew them and would bring a special sensitivity to the experience to co-officiate the ceremony. The first rabbi, from a liberal branch of Judaism, and mature in his pulpit experience delivered a homily in which he spoke of the Jewish tradition that matches were made in heaven. He went on to say that when marriages did not work out, it obviously means they were never meant to be. This marriage, he said, was in truth the one always meant to happen, the

6. Avot D'Rabbi Natan 14:6

one determined in heaven. The other, in each case, was never supposed to happen. The children, six of them, ranging in age from eight to twenty-one, were sitting among the guests. How cruel was it for them to have to listen to the rabbi's "loving" words in which he essentially made them a "mistake," since their mother and father were never by heaven supposed to have wed.

As if that were not enough, the second rabbi at the conclusion of the ceremony called on all the children, together with the new couple, to drink together from the "cup of blessing" over which the prayers were recited under the *chuppah*. He then proceeded to tell all of them that they were one family blessed with sweetness, unity and harmony. Now, I had seen the expression of several of the children during the ceremony. Two, in fact, at one point, walked out. In the rabbi's desire to use ritual to "make it right," he rode over the ambivalent and in some cases conflicted feelings of the children at this time in order to put the seal of blessing on the event. My guess is that some of the children felt as if they were drinking a cup of poison. How could one who sees the final death of their dream of a home with their mother and father not feel sadness, even though they may also feel hope? In both cases, the rabbis officiating at the wedding got caught up with the ideal and missed the persons present. In glorifying love and renewal they failed to experience the inner drama before them lived out in the life of a family filled with brokenness and unhealed wounds. The rabbis embraced the Torah with its transcendent beauty but missed identifying with the suffering attendant to the human condition, even amid joy.

It is not only the emphasis on the cultivation of the spiritual self that often causes rabbis and seminarians to miss persons in the mundane and flawed dimensions of their lives. The rabbi in his/her role is called upon to be a teacher. The teaching role is hierarchical. The Medrash understands the word "children" in the verse "And you shall teach them diligently to your children"[7] to refer not to biological children, but to one's students, who are one's

---

7. Deuteronomy 6:7

spiritual children.[8] Indeed the rabbi as teacher is seen as a parent bringing one to the next life even as one's natural parents brought him/her into this one. Parents relate to children from the one-up position. The teacher, as parent, is esteemed, respected as other, accorded honor that reflects the awareness of the inherent difference of status and accomplishment. It is an appropriate image for the rabbi to enter when giving a sermon, teaching a class, and in some counseling situations. But it is not the role the rabbi needs to apply when providing care. In his/her caring role, the rabbi needs to forsake the teacher/parent style of relating to the congregant as student/child, with its attendant distance, in order to become companion/friend to the hurting other. No sermons, lectures, pieces of wisdom belong to the bedside unless it is the patient in the bed giving them. Turning off the teacher/parent way of relating is not easy for rabbis. It engenders an uncomfortable, yet necessary sense of vulnerability. The rabbi needs to bring his/her "person" into his/her role and become unmasked, no small task.

Let me share a verbatim snippet of a rabbinical student who struggled to make the transition from teacher to companion so that we might see what the difference looks like.

Jacob was a third-year rabbinical student at Yeshiva University. He decided to take a summer unit of Clinical Pastoral Education to better prepare him for his career as a congregational rabbi. Over the course of the summer, Jacob was a full-time pastoral intern at Beth Israel Medical Center, where I was both director of the Pastoral Care and Education Department and supervisor of the CPE program. Jacob had several visits with Gloria, a sixty-year-old woman with metastasized breast cancer, and on one occasion with her husband, Max, who was present in the room. Jacob's goal was to help this woman to experience God's loving presence with her in her struggle by being a companion, validating Gloria's (and her husband's) suffering and helping her feel less alone.

In the first visit, Max engaged Jacob in a series of questions on themes ranging from the meaning of the names of God to the reason we no longer offer sacrifices. As Max grew more bold, he made

8. Sifri V'etchanan

his questions more personal.

Max: You know I want to speak to God and I don't understand why He doesn't answer me back. I told you how I went to synagogue…

Jacob: Yes, I remember.

Max: Well, God spoke to Abraham, Moses, why doesn't He speak to me?

Jacob: I suppose you have lots of questions for God.

Max: I sure do.

Jacob: What would you ask God?

Max: I'd ask Him why He's doing this to Gloria and me. But why doesn't He answer me?

Jacob: Well I don't know that God speaks as we humans speak. I am not even sure that's the way God spoke to the Patriarchs…

Max: I want Him to answer me. I don't see why I can't find out what's going on.

Jacob: I understand this must be confusing for you.

Max: Yes. I just want some info. I mean we must have done something to deserve this.

Jacob: Do you really think it works that way?

Max: Well, that's what it says, right?

Jacob: I don't know. Did you ever read the Book of Job?

Max: No, I want to know the answer. Is it there?

Jacob: Well Job was a righteous man and he began to suffer due to nothing he had done. It was part of a Divine… anyway. He had terrible troubles and his friends tried to tell him he had done something wrong and that now he was being punished by God. At the end of the book, Job loses it and finally cries out to God.

God answers from a whirlwind… So, in fact, although Job never really gets to understand why he suffered, he finds out he was righteous, no sin was the cause of his pain and suffering.

Max: Huh. Where is that in the Torah?

Jacob: Actually, it's in the last part of the Bible, in "Writings." Take a look at it.

Max: I will.

Jacob: I hear you're struggling. This has got to be so difficult.

Gloria: It is.

The visit concluded with the three of them, Jacob, Max and Gloria, reading a Psalm.

In the above visit, Jacob, as rabbi, found himself over and over again invited into the comfortable role of teacher. While he made good effort, particularly near the visit's close, to join with Max in his suffering, inevitably he could not resist the impulse to teach, with its attendant distance. Later that summer Jacob visited again. This time Max was not in the room. Jacob was intentional about getting down to be with Gloria and become her companion/friend. After some early pleasantries, it was clear Max wouldn't be there.

Jacob: So, can I bring up a chair and visit with you?

Gloria: Sure.

Jacob (pulls up a chair, moves a table, does some redecorating and finally has a place to sit down): So how are you doing?

Gloria: I'm doing all right. You know I found the prayer book you gave me last visit was very meaningful...pleading to God, having faith. I have a lot of Christian friends praying for me. They have so much faith...

Jacob: You have found it difficult to turn to God for strength?

Gloria: Well, yes, they just seem to have so much faith and they have a belief in the afterlife which they totally believe... Do we really have a view of an afterlife?

Jacob: Well, we believe in a "world to come," in which things will be different, better. Have you been thinking about these things a lot lately?

The visit continues in which Gloria shares some of her fears, her difficulties with her husband, and at times her anger with people who fail to appreciate her struggle. Jacob helps Gloria speak her heart with its confusion, avoiding opportunities to teach, instead choosing to understand so as to connect.

> Gloria: Anyway…I was talking to my cousin about all kinds of stuff. You know I have been thinking about holding my grandchild and how even if I get better I don't know if I'll ever be so well to do that. It's crazy, because I don't even have a grandchild.
>
> Jacob: Yes, but obviously the idea of doing that must be important to you!
>
> Gloria: Well, when there are things you imagined you would do one day…
>
> Jacob: It must be really hard for you to think about those things.
>
> Gloria: Yes, I guess we just hope, have faith. Boy if it were only as easy as my friends think it is.
>
> Jacob: Yes, I remember during our first visit we prayed together. Your request from God was so modest. Just a little more time.
>
> Gloria: That's all I want…

With the visit's close, Jacob prayed a spontaneous prayer capturing the yearning Gloria expressed and honoring their friendship.

In both of these visits Jacob was a rabbi to Gloria and Max. In the first visit he was rabbi as teacher. In the second he was rabbi as companion and shepherd. In the first visit Jacob answered questions. In the second Jacob explored the meaning the questions had so as to cultivate relationships. In the first visit the prayer was liturgical. In the second it was spontaneous, born out of the moment and the intimacy attained. In the first visit Jacob shared his wisdom. In the second he shared his heart. Caregiving is about sharing the heart. That is no small challenge for those whose lives have long been seen as an expression of their wisdom.

In truth the rabbi as caregiver needs not only to overcome his/ her own role image and the position that offers him/her most comfort. The rabbi must avoid the projections and expectations of those he/she serves. Men and women strive to find heroes. If there are none to be found, they are then invented. Much has been written in psychoanalytic literature, and in particular by Ernest Becker, in *The Denial of Death*, which helps us to understand the human need to idealize the imperfect.[9] In a world in which we feel unsafe and afraid, projecting gifts on another, even gifts totally not present in him/her, helps us to feel more secure and protected. We bestow attributes and competencies on those in positions of authority rather than face the anxiety of our finitude. The cost of that process is in the limitations it puts on our own emotional/ spiritual maturation.

The rabbi is a prime candidate for the idealized projections. In seeing him/her as saintly, wise, caring, and mature, we feel safe as his/her charge. It does not matter what the truth of the rabbi's personal life and development may be, we don't see it. And if circumstances compel us to see the rabbi's flaws, as in the event of a mistake made public, a family issue becomes known, or a limitation too glaring to conceal, the rabbi's downfall is swift and severe. Mistakes become moral weaknesses, family issues become scandals and limitations are seen as expressions of corruption. We cannot endure our hero's clay feet. We experience his/her shortcomings as betrayal. The fall is as quick as the rise. Neither reflects anything more than the drama of the "false god" doomed to disappoint.

In times of illness when the world feels ever more unsafe than usual, for many the yearning for the all-wise, all-good rabbi becomes even greater. The sick and suffering want someone to say "it's OK," or better still, "you're OK." They want to identify with those who offer protection real or imagined. When the rabbi enters the room, the patient wants a teacher, a mentor, the one who knows. Max, in the verbatim snippet above, wanted Jacob to be the repository of wisdom. His questions belie his need to have for himself someone who knows the answers and with whom he

9. Ernest Becker, *The Denial of Death*, (New York, Free Press, 1975)

can be in relationship, even more than his need for the answers themselves. And yet, as Jacob came to realize, he could not be the protective presence Max sought. Nor should he be if Max and Gloria are to live this story and make meaning for themselves from it. Indeed the mature caregiver, whether he/she be clergy or other, needs to resist playing into the role of the idealized savior/protector. He/she needs to have the wisdom to recognize that while accepting the projections from the ones in the bed may offer some immediate gratification to them and even satisfy his/her own longing to be loved, it ultimately keeps persons from the growth opportunity these times of travail provide. It infantilizes them. It sustains a lie at a time when confronting truth is the ultimate responsibility.

The measure of whether good care was provided cannot be determined on the basis of a satisfied consumer. Too often I hear patients rave about a caregiver who simply offered them empty clichés and never bothered to even hear their story. Yes, they may have felt better after the visit, but healing is not about feeling better but about feeling more oneself, more authentic, more truly alive. That occurs in the context of relationship. It occurs when the rabbi, like Jacob, resonates with Gloria, rather than answers Max, as in the verbatim snippets above.

How does the rabbi as caregiver go about avoiding the projections of his/her patients/congregants? In a classic work on healing relationship, *The Transparent Self*, Sidney M. Jourard challenges the notion of helping by being unknown. On the contrary, he argues, one needs to let oneself be known in order to make the other feel safe enough to reveal him/herself. He calls for mutual self-disclosure with the goal of engendering trust as the risks are shared.[10] While surely rabbis have every reason to feel hesitant about self-disclosure, unless the rabbi is willing to make him/herself known as a person with his/her own limitations, idealizations will abound. To be in relationship implies a mutuality. While the patient/congregant may not need to know his/her rabbi's/chaplain's every flaw, he/she needs to see the rabbi/chaplain as a person, father, mother,

---

10. Sidney M. Jourard, *The Transparent Self* (New York, Van Nostrand, 1971)

husband, wife, and so on. If Jacob in our earlier verbatim snippet with Max had said, "You know at times I too wonder where God is and why He doesn't talk to me when I most need God," in response to Max's question on why God does not talk to him, their relationship might have taken a different turn. Max would have had to confront Jacob as a fellow traveler on life's, at times, painful journey. They could become companions in seeking faith amid unfairness. True, Max in his yearning for the quick fix might have resisted the invitation to a new relationship. But is not that what the rabbi/chaplain needs to offer, the chance for spiritual maturation in response to challenge!

The odyssey of the rabbi as he/she moves from the role he/she is most prepared for in the rabbinate to that of caregiver is complex and challenging. The rabbi must lead by forgoing his/her identification with the spiritual and ideal to identify with the earthy and the broken within. He/she must surrender the position of teacher with its attendant distance and instead become a companion. He/she must risk becoming a person, warts and all, to successfully enter into relationship in which the idealization of the rabbi is surrendered for the gift of the acquisition of spiritual maturation for oneself. With all that it takes, is it any wonder that so few rabbis are in fact good at building healing relationships? Moreover, is it any wonder that so few rabbis can say of their congregations that they have grown, not necessarily in members, or in budget, but in spiritual maturity under their leadership? Indeed, as rabbis are enabled to become effective caregivers, they not only relieve suffering, they become instruments through which the Jewish community attains new levels of spiritual maturation, and becomes more spiritually adult.

Chapter 5
Finding God at the Bedside

My God, my God,
> why have You abandoned me
> why so far from delivering me
> and from my anguished roaring.

My God,
> I cry by day – You answer not;
> by night, and have no respite.[1]

At the deepest level our suffering is an experience of the abandonment of the Divine. More than all the individual aspects related to any loss, no matter how great they may be, is the suffering rooted in the sense that God has rejected us or, still worse, chosen to persecute us without reason. Over and over in the Book of Job, God is challenged not for the horrific afflictions Job is made to suffer, nor for the circumstances he is forced to endure. Rather Job's core lament is "For the arrows of the Almighty are in me; my spirit drinks their poison; God's terrors are arrayed against me."[2]

We have already described in considerable detail in Chapter Two the core element of suffering as one of estrangement. In illness and in loss, we become disconnected from our sense of self in all its manifestations. Inasmuch as the essence of our self from a

1. Psalms 22:2-3
2. Job 6:4

spiritual vantage point is the Godly soul implanted in us, the estrangement from that soul is experienced as an estrangement from God. We may utter prayers to God but we struggle to feel God's presence. Relationship is absent. The aloneness from God makes the experience of suffering most difficult to endure. As a great Hassidic Master once said, "I can endure, O God, any travail, if only I could know I was enduring it for You." Job's experience of the presence of the Divine in the whirlwind does not resolve his questions or explain his plight, and yet it is enough. Knowing God has not forsaken him makes for all the relief he needs.

We need to understand the question often posed by patients, "What have I done to deserve this?" in this context. Frequently, the caregiver is quick to respond by sharing a theology designed to free the sick and suffering from the additional burden of a sense of guilt to compound their situation. The caregiver, hoping to remove the sense of responsibility from the one in the bed or his/her family, will suggest that God is not a punitive parent and suffering does not need to imply wrongdoing. What the caregiver may not realize is that frequently the sense of being punished for sin, if one could be identified, would bring relief to patients and families. At least then they would know their suffering had meaning. God, even if disciplining them, was in relationship with them. They were not abandoned. On the other hand, to the extent that suffering goes unrelated to God-human affairs, the ones enduring it feel alienated and alone in a world they cannot fathom and with a God who does not care. That from a spiritual perspective leads to the depression so commonly found among those enduring long-term stories of suffering and loss.

The same needs to be realized when providing care for a patient/family where we expect anger to be present. At times the chaplain or rabbi seeks to offer support by encouraging the suffering to express their anger. We may point out to them that anger is an acceptable religious response, and that in expressing our anger, in particular at God, we free ourselves up to engage God with greater authenticity. What may not be realized is that the hesitancy to get angry is not our concern about its justification or even its acceptance as appropriate religious conduct. What may be motivating the reticence to voice anger is fear, fear that the anger, while justified and acceptable, may further distance the already hidden God. The cost of the honest expression of feelings is just too great to bear. It is not theological lectures patients and families require to be honest with God in the fullness of their experiences. What they need is the trust that in doing so God will stay with them.

And yet the question remains, Where is God in the midst of suffering? Nowhere is that issue more poignantly raised than in a story from Elie Wiesel's *Night*.

When the labor force returned to camp, they saw three gallows set up. The three ill-fated to be hanged were in chains. One was a young boy.

It was not a simple matter for the SS to hang a young boy in front of a large crowd. Even the *Lagerkapo* refused to be the executioner.

The three condemned stood together on chairs, and nooses were tightened around their necks.

"Long live liberty!" cried the two adults.

But the boy was silent.

"Where is God? Where is He?" someone behind Wiesel asked.

Then the signal to pull the chairs came.

Then the march past the gallows began. The two adults were no longer living.

But the young boy was still alive. Being so light, the agony of his death carried on for more than half an hour.

"And we had to look him full in the face. He was still alive when I passed in front of him. His tongue was still red, his eyes not yet glazed," Wiesel recalled.

"Where is God now?" the same voice asked.

And I heard a voice within me answer him: Where is He? Here He is – He is hanging here on this gallows…"[3]

---

3. Elie Wiesel, *Night* (New York, Avon Books, 1960) pp 74-76

The caregiver, one who enters into a deep empathic relationship with the suffering must indeed have the same question in circumstances, if less dramatic, no less real. Every time a child dies, leukemia attacks a young father, a mother is stricken with breast cancer, a senior has a stroke, the question is present if only we look the suffering in the eyes. If we, like Wiesel, are present with the suffering, "Where is God?" is not a theological problem but a crisis of faith and relationship.

However, there is another side to the story, one equally compelling. Those of us who have been fortunate enough to be present to others in the midst of their crisis and travail have at times known a most sacred spiritual moment, precisely in the depth of the others' anguish.

I can remember visiting with Miriam, a fifty-four-year-old woman racked with pain caused by a metastasized cancer ravishing her body. Miriam challenged me over and over in my visits with her, "Where is God?" "How could He do this to me?" I felt the enormous unfairness of Miriam's predicament. I heard her angst. And yet in the very moment she felt God's abandonment and betrayal, I felt a sacred spirituality, a holy presence I could not quite explain to myself and certainly would not attempt to explain to Miriam.

Even in reading Wiesel's account of the horrific injustice done to the child above, as we take it in, shed a tear, and feel the outrage, we encounter a certain inexplicable spiritual stirring, an awareness of the holy within. I have often thought to answer the question "Where is God?" in that episode, God was in the conscience of the questioner, in Wiesel, in the tears they shed and in their outrage.

The presence of the spiritual in the world of the suffering is complex. The Torah is quite clear. God, in meting out Israel's punishment, will absent God's self from them.

God tells Moses near the end of Deuteronomy that in response to Israel's forsaking of the Covenant and embracing false gods, "Then My anger will flare up against them. I will abandon them and hide My countenance from them."[4]

And later in the same verse, "And they shall say on that day,

---

4. Deuteronomy 31:17

surely it is because our God is not in our midst that these evils have befallen us."[5] Later Jewish theologians have referred to this as the "Eclipse of God" in the midst of suffering.[6]

But the Talmud presents a perspective quite different. "Rabbi Shimon Bar Yochai said, 'Come and see how precious Israel is to the Holy One Blessed Be He that every place to which they were exiled the *Shekhina* went with them'."[7] He then went on to demonstrate by reference to scriptural passages that in all the exiles from Egypt to Babylon and to everywhere in the future where the *Galut* may lead, God's *Shekhina* is with Israel. How do we reconcile the Torah passage confirming God's absence with the Talmudic teachings insisting on God's presence?

A similar conundrum exists when we look for sources relative to the suffering of individuals. We opened this chapter referencing the passage from Psalms in which suffering is experienced as God's abandonment. Yet the Talmud teaches that God is not only not absent to the sick, but more present with them. "Rabbi Avin said in the name of Rav, 'Whence do we know that the *Shekhina* resides above the bed of the sick...from the verse The Lord sustains me[8]'."[9] And still later in that same portion of the Talmud the rabbis understood the idea of the presence of the *Shekhina* with the sick as having *halachic* implications: "One who visits the sick should not sit on the bed nor on a chair or bench. Rather one should wrap oneself and sit on the ground for the *Shekhina* is above the bed of one who is ill."[10] Again, as in the case of Israel's suffering, we are left to understand how it is that God is most present when the sufferer feels God's abandonment.

The answer, I suggest, is that indeed God is more present in times of suffering than in the routine of life. God loves us. In our pain and danger, God is drawn to us by God's love and compassion.

---

5. Deuteronomy 31:17

6. Martin Buber, *Eclipse of God* (New York, Harper 1952)

7. Megilah 29a

8. Psalms 41:4

9. Nedarim 40:7

10. Nedarim 40b

It is for this reason we are mandated to be ourselves, present to the suffering in the first place, as the rabbis charged us to the *mitzvah* of *bikur cholim* and *nichum aveilim* out of the imperative of *imitatio Dei*, even as we discussed in our first chapter. The experience of abandonment given voice to by the Psalmist and expressed in the national drama in the verses of Deuteronomy are true to the way the suffering encounter their moment. In the awfulness of the pain, fear and aloneness, the suffering become enveloped by their circumstances. They lose the capacity to feel the Divine in their midst. It is their finitude that the suffering most sense, not their transcendence, be it in family, community, God or self. This is the very estrangement that is at the core of suffering, as we discussed in great detail in Chapter Two.

In truth, however, God is most present when we are most hurting. And yet we cannot access God directly due to our limited horizon and disorientation from our spiritual selves. There is but one way for us when we are in the midst of suffering to encounter the holy. And here lies the great truth. We encounter the holy in our suffering through the eyes and presence of the witness. It is through the witness, the one entering the room of the sick and the suffering that God's presence is made known to them. In identifying with the suffering and their circumstances, and yet remaining another, the witness feels the presence of the sacred and mirrors it back to the suffering in the bed. Indeed it is through the intermediary that when we suffer we may yet know God in our midst and feel God's love. Let me explain.

I remember making a visit to a Jewish man, a member of the community where I served as rabbi, but not a member of my congregation. The visit was meaningful as together we explored the man's hopes and fears. We prayed together a spontaneous prayer at the visit's close. On my way out, the man's private-duty nurse, who had been present throughout the visit, asked if she could speak to me a moment. When outside the room, she proceeded to tell me, "Rabbi, you should know, when you go into a room, you don't go in alone." I thought about her remark for some time. Originally it made me feel wonderful. "Wow," I thought, "this woman experienced God with me in my visit." But on reflection, as nice as it was to think that way, it didn't ring true. Yes, I, too, experienced something sacred in the room, but I would be hard-pressed to say its source inhered in me. After all, I didn't have a prevailing spiritual sense about me when I entered the room, and any inspiration I carried out the door left not long after the visit. Where did the sense of the holy she experienced as a witness to the visit come from?

If I am to believe the sources in my tradition discussed above, I dare say the sacred presence felt in that visit was there already in the room before I arrived. The *Shekhina* was indeed hovering over the sick man's bed. If I did anything it was that I allowed myself to catch the Divine presence. I put myself in position to feel the imminent God. In listening to the man and the integrity of his struggle, I experienced more than an individual fighting to survive the moment; I sensed the sacred drama of the human yearning for hope, meaning and faith. I saw this man's story in the larger context and in that validated its holiness, the holiness present in the struggle, indeed the holiness of the *Shekhina*. Precisely because I both identified with the man in the depth of his circumstances and yet maintained an otherness through which I remained centered, I could see what he could not, feel that which was beyond him. In my words, through my demeanor, by dint of the respect for the holy ground I was on evident in me, the man could gain access to the presence of God he, on his own, felt detached from. I did as the Talmud mandated. I wrapped myself and symbolically sat on the ground before the *Shekhina* above his bed. He experienced God as present in me, in my presence, as did the private duty nurse. In truth, God's presence was there in response to him, and out of God's love for him, and God's partnership in his drama.

My pastoral visit with Miriam, discussed earlier, reflected the same dynamics. Miriam was so devastated by her pain and so caught up with the unhappiness of it all that she lost contact with the spiritual drama in which she was the major player. In living the story, she could not get the distance from it to appreciate the experience as full with meaning and theological import. Yes, her story was sad, even tragic, but Miriam's struggle was not by any means empty. In being present with her and in a deep way engaging the drama, albeit with the distance of another, I could encounter the awesomeness of this woman affirming, "There must be a reason." "There must be justice." It was in her relentless commitment, despite it all, that life and death cannot simply be random and that the human experience cannot be devoid of meaning that the very God she yearned to experience could be seen in her and felt in her presence.

In truth, though I felt a special sacredness present in my visit with Miriam I could not successfully get her to experience it. The idea of witnessing is not the same as teaching. Telling another that God is present for them provides them information they may choose to believe or not. But that does not get them to experience that presence as their own. It is by evidencing the presence of the holy in one's speech, manner and mood that the one in the bed feels the presence of the holy. It is through the spiritual inspiration as evident in the one offering care and relationship with the sufferer that the suffering come to know the experience of holiness for themselves. Miriam was too overwhelmed to enter with me into the relationship that might have allowed her to feel the presence of the God she so desperately sought. Try as I might to build a rapport, she had too much pain to do more than moan and lament. She was not able to feel the presence of God. She was unable in her circumstances to even see and feel my presence as more than a body in the room. Tragically, she remained isolated and alone.

In the sad and tragic story told by Wiesel and referenced earlier, it was not only the boy who was hung who likely felt the absence of God, but there, even the observers asked "Where is God?" In being present to that tragedy they were too close to see anything but overwhelming horror. It was not only the boy's experience they were living, but their own as well. They had not the distance necessary to be witnesses and to see the event as a profound spiritual drama. They could not see their own poignant expression of the yearning for the Divine in the midst of unmitigated evil as a manifestation of sublime spiritual significance. They could not experience

God's pained silence in the face of bold avarice and murder as itself filling the moment with a transcendence and awe. All that was left to us, we who read the story, we who have the distance necessary to witness. For us the very questions "Where is God?", "Where is God now?" are filled with a haunting spirituality.

In light of the above, it becomes understandable why family members while frequently providing excellent care to their ill and suffering loved ones are rarely able to serve as conduits to help engender a sense of the holy or the meaningful. It is precisely because they are too close and because the story of suffering belongs to them as well that they typically lack the distance necessary to serve as witnesses to the larger spiritual drama unfolding before their eyes. It remains for others, chaplains, rabbis, friends, those who choose to enter the depth of the experience, and for whom the story is poignant and compelling, but not their own, who can be true witnesses, and offer a gateway to an awareness of the Divine for both the patient and his/her family alike.

The laws attendant to visiting the sick make clear that the visitor, be he/she a rabbi or other, has not done his/her *mitzvah* unless he/she has prayed for the patient.[11] While some may consider it sufficient to put off the prayer at the bedside until a more formal occasion arises, say on Monday or Thursday at services in the synagogue when the Torah is read and the *mishebairach* for the sick is recited, that is not in keeping with the purpose of the visitor's prayer. In fact, there is a teaching in tradition rooted in scriptural passages that "greater is the power of prayer said for oneself than prayer recited by another on one's behalf."[12] In fact, the rabbis wanted the visitors to pray at the bedside of the sick, where the *Shekhina* already is present, so as to arouse the motivation of the sick to pray for themselves. The rabbis understood that prayer was a difficult experience for the suffering. Oh yes, they might lament; they might moan. But prayer as a plaintive encounter with the Divine is most often too difficult when one is feeling God's absence. The visitor, as we discussed, can access the holy in the sufferer's

---

11. Shulchan Aruch, Yoreh Deah 335:4

12. Braishit Rabah, Vayerah 53:14

milieu. The visitor is the witness to the presence of the *Shekhina* to which the sufferer is blind. When he/she prays at the bedside out of that heightened sense of the sacredness in this place and time, it can serve to motivate the suffering themselves, awaken them and their slumbering spiritual senses. In the end, it is not the prayer of the visitor that is most called for. The visitor's prayers need to be experienced as a key to unlock the profound and heartfelt prayers sequestered in the heart of the sick and suffering themselves.

Witnessing the holy at the bedside is a deeply moving experience. When we as caregivers are open to the encounter it has the capacity to transform us. We know an immediacy to the Divine unparalleled in ordinary life. In knowing the other in the depths of his/her suffering, we glimpse the spirit of God. For many who do this work, that is all the reward they ask for. They are drawn time and time again into the midst of another's hell because indeed there they can find an intimacy with the holy otherwise inaccessible. Those who enter the world of the suffering focused on fixing and helping, those who fail to join their brothers and sisters in their story of hurt and confusion, will never know this precious presence. Too busy giving advice, moralizing, or avoiding the woundedness before them, they are cheated as much as the suffering from a redemptive moment. When those who fix and help at the bedside feel good after a visit it is all about the ego and its preservation. When those who witness feel good after a visit it is because they indeed have rendezvoused with the sacred.

Chapter 6
Spiritual Assessment

> *One of the great Hassidic Masters said to his Hassidim, "I have learned the meaning of love from witnessing two Polish peasants in a local tavern. They were drinking together and obviously enjoying each other's company immensely. Finally I overheard one say to the other, 'Jan, I love you.' To which Jan responded, 'If you really love me, tell me where I hurt.'"*

To be an effective caregiver and fulfill the Torah imperative challenging us to this work of *hesed*, "Love thy neighbor as thyself"[1], we need to know where the other is hurting. We must understand the hurt, its locus, its quality, its story. In truth, we cannot really know the hurt of another unless we know him/her in the context of his/her life. To know a person in his/her state of suffering, we must have a sense of what wellness looks like for this person. All too often we enter the scene and assume incorrectly that our entry point, and the experience we learn of at that moment, is the place in which the other is living.

Let me share a personal experience that may help clarify the point. In my own life I had gone through a painful divorce. I had worked for several years to reclaim my sense of wholeness even amid the brokenness and to affirm the meaning of that which remained even after the loss. I had moved through a long and difficult passage in which the prevailing sadness had been over time

1. Leviticus 19:18

redirected into a sense of pride for that which had been achieved both in the years of marriage and in the aftermath. While working at the New York University Medical Center as a chaplain, I came across a friend of many years prior, who was there visiting with his sick father. In renewing our relationship, we asked about each other's lives. Upon hearing my story, his response was as predictable as it was unsettling. He asked, "Are you married?" I told him that I was divorced. He said, "Oy vay." He asked, "Any children?" I said five. He responded, "Oh how awful." In truth, if I was living the divorce in its first moments, if it was news for me, as it was for him, I might have had the same reaction. Marriage, divorce, children – a tragedy indeed! He no doubt thought he was being empathic. In fact, he was expressing feelings that did not match mine at all in that moment. I was grateful for my children, and each was a blessing. What was for him a story of sadness was now for me a story of deliverance.

Caregivers make the mistake frequently of relating to the story told to them rather than to the person sharing it. The sick and/or suffering may share a vignette from their past that we who hear it for the first time find almost overwhelming. It may be a story that transpired fifty years ago, yet for us it is new. We react to the story by bringing the person sharing it back to that place and time as if we could provide pastoral care retroactively. What we miss is that the storyteller in sharing their past is more likely not asking us to go back on history long since processed. Rather, the storyteller is asking us to see how the story of the past has somehow become important to him/her here and now, in his/her current circumstances. The task of the caregiver is to feel for the fullness of the person so as to discern the meaning his/her sharing has in the context of his/her predicament.

The work we are calling for here is one of assessment. In order to enter into a healing relationship, we must first spend time making an assessment of the other person in terms of his/her life, hopes, disappointments, triumphs and losses. If, as we have described in Chapter Three, the goal of our care is to help restore the person suffering to him/herself, we must be open to discover what that self might look like. Wellness of a spiritual nature will not look the same to me as it does to you. When I am well I may be profoundly in touch with my emotions and expressive of my spirit through them. Wellness for you may be in expressing acute intellectual capacity and the enhanced motivation to study.

The idea of assessing the person being cared for is consistent with the concept, rooted in tradition, that every malady suffered has an impact on the wellness of the spirit as well as the body. In the language of the liturgical *mishebairach*, the prayer for the sick recited in synagogue, we mention the name of the person ill and then go on to ask for his/her healing of *guf*, body, and *nefesh*, spirit. It makes no difference whether the person being prayed for has metastasized cancer or a broken leg. In all cases, when one is sick one needs a healing of both body and spirit, for indeed both willy-nilly have been made ill. The illness of the *guf* is a matter to be determined by physicians. They have a language to identify both the symptoms and its causes. The illness of the spirit must be diagnosed by competent caregivers. They must have a language both for the identification of symptoms and for the discernment of the root issues.

We must be clear when we write of symptoms and root issues for the illness of the *nefesh*. I am not referring to the reasons why a person became ill. It is not the etiology of the spiritual malady that we dare attempt to identify. God's ways are inscrutable, and any lessons learned belong to the sick themselves to identify. It no more belongs to the caregivers to name the spiritual reason for a person's suffering than for the physician to lay cause of his/her physical circumstances. Rather, the challenge for the caregiver is to discern, in the here and now, what are the natures of the spiritual issues impacting those who are sick and infirmed and give them coherent expression. In the realm of physical illness, words such as tumor, inflammation, infection, and blockage become relevant descriptive language. In the assessment of the spiritual malady attendant to illness, we might utilize words such as despair, alienation, meaninglessness, and fear. All of these terms have a connection to affairs of the spirit. I did not use words such as depression, anxiety, and withdrawal, which might more commonly be found in a psychiatric assessment. Indeed, in saying all illness affects the spirit as well as the body, we are not raising psychiatric concerns, though they may, on occasion, be present. We are not concerned with pathology. We are rather concerned with the person's divergence from the spiritual balance that is most associated with well-being for him/her.

Much has been written concerning spiritual assessment in pastoral care literature over the past several years. The Joint Commission on Accreditation of Healthcare Organizations (JCAHO), accrediting both medical institutions and geriatric facilities, has come to expect documented spiritual assessment as a reliable indicator insuring that the patient's/resident's needs are being met. Many models for spiritual assessment are available to the reader. For my part, I believe spiritual assessment must start with determining what a person who is ill and suffering needs to be whole. What are the ingredients that constitute a sense of well-being. While, even as discussed earlier, individuals will differ on what wholeness will look like for them, all persons share basic needs. It is the extent of each need, and the ways these key needs express themselves in individual's lives, that may vary and makes for the uniqueness of persons.

The spiritual needs are rooted in four foundational concerns. First, the sick and suffering need to feel affirmed. That is, they need to feel that even with their physical struggles they remain OK as persons. Illness may have compromised their body but they are no less whole than they were prior to its onset. Second, the sick and suffering need to feel valued. That is, they need to know that even with their situation they remain vital members of society with a role and a purpose that makes them important to the lives of others. Indeed, they need to feel that they are deserving of drawing on life's resources as much now as when they were well. Third, the ill and suffering need to feel secure. They need to have a sense of safety amid the turmoil in their situation. They need to find an anchor in the prevailing storm. Fourth, the ill and suffering need to feel they belong. That is, they need to have a sense that despite the experiences of isolation attached to their struggle they are not alone. Others are with them in community even when not always present. In the remainder of this chapter, we will explore each of these four themes – affirmation, value, security, and belonging – in greater detail. We will explicate the struggle, identify what each looks like when present in caregiving conversation with the sick and suffering, and develop strategies that offer meaningful response.

The Need to Feel Affirmed

When we are sick, when our bodies are malfunctioning, it is common to experience a sense of inner diminishment. Typically, when sick we loathe ourselves. We, at times, even feel ashamed of our circumstances. Moreover, we are often ashamed of the feelings we have around those circumstances, ashamed of the fear, ashamed of the worry, ashamed of the shame itself. So much of the suffering attached to illness and loss is located in the depleted self-esteem. So much of the work of healing is to facilitate a renewal of the sufferer's sense of inner goodness and worth.

Let me share a portion of a verbatim account of a visit with you where the dominant spiritual issue is reflective of this struggle for self-esteem in the midst of illness. Mr. L. was a seventy-three-year-old man recovering from a recent stroke. He was a European refugee who the chaplain, in earlier visits, had identified as "the strong silent type."

C1: Mr. L. It's Rabbi P. again. How are you doing?
P1: OK.

C2: Mind if I sit down? (P does not look at C; he shrugs.)
Are you waiting for them to take you somewhere?
P2: Always going somewhere. Just came back.

C3: From physical therapy? Occupational therapy?
P3: Physical therapy.

C4: What are they working on?

P4: Working on?

C5: What are they exercising with you?

P5: My right hand. I can do nothing with my right hand, and now I can lift it a little. (P lifts hand about two inches.)

C6: That's an improvement.... Last week your hand was in your lap.... It means you are getting better.

P6: It's like I'm a child, nothing...I can hold nothing. What's the point?

The patient went on to lament his situation and to doubt himself even more than the severity of his condition.

In the above vignette, the chaplain attempted to respond to what he heard as Mr. L.'s disappointments. Like Debbie's mother in Chapter One, he hoped to restore Mr. L. by fixing his perception about his circumstances. The efforts he made toward that end go nowhere. Mr. L. cannot be lifted out of his doldrums until he can accept himself and bless who he is even with his paralysis. What kind of intervention might in fact raise self-esteem and help Mr. L. affirm himself even in his physically compromised state?

There is a wonderful story of the Rebbe from Kotzk, a Hassidic Master known for his relentless pursuit of truth. A disciple told him his woes.

"I come from Rizhin. There everything is simple, everything is clear. I prayed and I knew I was praying; I studied and I knew I was studying. Here in Kotzk everything is mixed up and confused – I suffer from it, Rebbe. Terribly. I am lost. Please help me so I can pray and study as before. Please help me to stop suffering."

The Rebbe smiled at his disciple in tears and asked: "And who told you that God is interested in your studies and your prayers? And what if He prefers your tears and suffering?"

The Rebbe's strategy in the story above is effective precisely because he does not minimize the tears and the confusion of his disciple. He does not try to deny his disciple's experience or its validity. On the contrary, the Rebbe validates the disciple's experience. He makes all the disciple's feelings not reasons for shame, but reasons for pride.

The chaplain in the case presented with Mr. L. does not have the authority or the relationship with Mr. L. to intervene as the Rebbe did. And yet the chaplain, too, came to realize that Mr. L.'s need for self-affirmation was the major spiritual issue requiring a response. He changed direction in the conversation and rather than attempt to fix the situation he chose to give Mr. L. a chance to reclaim his larger self beyond the current context and its heaviness.

> C15: Are you retired now?
> P15: Yeah...two years ago.
>
> C16: What did you do?
> P16: (For the first time he turned his chair to look at the chaplain.) I was in tool and dye....Owned my own shop.
>
> C17: Where was it?
> P17: In Dearborn. Lived there too...with the goyim and everything.

The chaplain went on to hear Mr. L.'s story as he experienced renewed self-importance. By the end of the visit, Mr. L. was no longer reactive to the chaplain's questions. He had seized hold of the visit, made closure, and validated the visit's meaning. The chaplain, like the Rebbe, offered most of all a loving acknowledgment of the suffering of the other. Rather than minimize the feelings of the disciple and Mr. L., in each case an effort was made to honor the person as true, and yet not necessarily go along with the concomitant self-diminishment each experienced.

The Need to Feel Valued

No one enjoys being the recipient of charity for very long. Each of us needs to feel our journey has meaning. As has often been quoted, "One can endure any suffering as long as he/she has a reason why." Many people's suffering is not rooted in their physical distress, but in an emptiness founded in a failure to see their circumstances as purposeful. When patients ask, "Why is this happening to me?" "Why is God doing this to me?" frequently they are not looking for reasons. They are looking for meaning. The story is told of Rabbi Levi Yitzchak of Berditchev:

> "One Passover eve, tortured by the mystery of collective suffering and evil, the rabbi burst out pleading: "Tonight we celebrate our Exodus from Egypt. According to tradition, four sons question the father on the meaning of the event. No, not four, only three. The fourth does not even know the question. I am this fourth. Not that I lack questions, Lord. But I don't know how to put them. Anyhow, even if I knew I wouldn't dare. And so I don't ask You why we are persecuted and massacred in every place and under every pretext, but I would at least like to know whether all our suffering is for You."

Let me share a verbatim account of a visit where this spiritual concern, the need to feel valued, is the prominent issue. Jack is an eighty-two-year-old married man, the father of three sons and grandfather of eight. He had a successful career in manufacturing. In fact, he owned five plants. He was wealthy and charitable and active in the Jewish community. In this verbatim account, Jack, who was in the hospital, summoned the rabbi because he wanted to make funeral arrangements. On entering the room, the rabbi was confused. Jack, while indeed lying in bed in a hospital room, appeared vigorous and showed anything but the physical appearance of a person at death's door. Also present was Jack's oldest son. We pick up the visit when it turned to the current situation.

S1: So why aren't you fighting for life, Dad?

P1: Tell him rabbi. Tell him to let me die.

C1: Jack, you look better than you did when I was here last week. Why do you want to die?

P2: *Et tu, Brute?* Because I have nothing to live for. I can't walk, I can hardly move and I can't get out of bed.

S2: But he's getting stronger....You lifted your legs.... Tell him.

C2: Is it true? Are you getting stronger? (Patient went on to confirm his physical improvement. He nevertheless reaffirmed his desire to die.)

C3: Your sons all want you to stick around. The people who work with you, too. It seems you have a lot of quality in your life. Isn't there?

P3: Yeah…but they pity me. They don't need me.

C4: What about your grandchildren?

P4: They don't need me…but that's the reason I haven't jumped out the window. They are the best. They're beautiful and bright and most of all they love me as much as I love them, which is a lot. I didn't want their last memory of me to be suicide.

It's important to note that Jack, in this visit, is clear that he feels loved. He realizes that his children, his grandchildren, even his rabbi care for him deeply. Yet it is not enough. He has no work to do. He feels no one needs him. Unlike Mr. L. in the earlier verbatim, Jack accepts himself. He may even love himself. But he cannot endure a life if it is not expressive of meaning, and fused with the opportunity to contribute to the lives of others.

When a person is experiencing a diminished sense of value, the last thing he/she needs is someone who says he/she is valuable. The very reliance on the other to foster that message compromises the sense of feeling useful the sufferer requires. While well intentioned, all the interventions of both the son and the rabbi in the visit above are more likely to strengthen Jack's sense of being the object of pity rather than turn him around. Caregiving, as one of my students once observed, is about "showing, not telling." To help Jack find meaning, Jack would need to experience a sense of purpose in the here and now, become teacher to the rabbi, mentor to his son. To restore Jack to a place of spiritual balance, where he once again could sense meaning in his life, the rabbi's best response would be to partner with Jack, allow Jack to use himself to help the rabbi in the context of their meeting. Jack needs opportunities to give, not receive. The caregiver must be creative in presenting these opportunities.

It is for the reason of allowing the one who is ill to give that I encourage caregivers not to decline the kindness extended to them by patients and others receiving care. When the person visited asks you to have a cookie, a fruit, a cup of tea (in the case of a home visit), accept it. In accepting the favor of the suffering, we grant them perhaps the gift they require most. We make it possible for them to feel valued and needed. No matter if the food is not kosher. Save it and discard it later. No matter if you are not hungry. Take it and give the other the satisfaction. Just as the caregiver needs to give, so, too, does the recipient of care. Illness often robs the sick, most of all, of their sense of being benefactors to others and thereby deserving their place in the world.

The Need to Feel Secure

We need to be able to count on certain conditions as stable and rooted. The moment we begin to doubt the reliability of our anchors, say in family or job, we become anxious. That anxiety can have debilitating consequences beyond the realization of our worst fears. In our anxiety, we can become paralyzed, lose ourselves, recede into despair. When we experience the change of circumstances common to the onset of illness and loss, something we relied on has been compromised. As much as our bodies have been affected so, too, have our psyches been bruised. We often develop a heightened sense of fear, fear for the future, fear that we will be engulfed in a world out of our control, with its consequences too scary to consider. When rabbis, chaplains, friends, and/or family visit the suffering it is the fear they often first encounter. At times the fear is palpable. The patient suffering fidgets nervously, communicates anxiety in his/her voice and manner. More often the fear is less obvious. It is embarrassing to admit being afraid, and what's more, it is assumed acknowledging the fear will make it worse. Typically, when the sick and suffering are afraid, they become more silent, withdrawn, hidden. They present a stoicism that masks the terror within. Perhaps they may try to distance themselves by watching television or listening to music, neither of which they can focus on or enjoy. Oh but the nights, those times when the insides churn with no relief. Those times can be devastating, sleepless, unbearable.

The tendency to protect the vulnerability experienced in fear often shows up in fear's shadow expression, anger. Fear and anger are responses to the same irritation, the unsettledness of life, its upheaval and unpredictability. When the suffering get angry, often it is a variation on fear, a response to feeling out of control. If we can get past the blowing winds, we will often discover the insecurities lying within. Let's look at the case of Lois, a sixty-year-old married woman with uterine cancer that had spread to her small intestine. After battling the cancer for better than a year, the doctors informed her she would need a colostomy. Her rabbi came to visit at the request of Lois's son, who informed the rabbi that she was depressed.

P1: Oh rabbi, it's so nice of you to come see me. How did you hear?
C1: The boys told me.

P2: I hate it. I hate it. It's bad enough I have no hair. All my femininity is gone. I can take that. But now I can't even go to the bathroom normally.
C2: Lois, Lois…you're angry aren't you?

P3: I don't show it to my children. I hate when I complain. But I can't take it anymore.

C3: Lois, are you angry at the cancer or that you're losing things we all take for granted?

P4: Both! And more...I'm so angry at so much... (Lois went on to describe her anger with her husband, who she felt complained about problems so trivial relative to hers.)

P5: Oh God, I just feel they don't understand. They don't see what they do. I don't have pain, thank God, and I still do all the things that I did – I just don't feel right.

Lois manifested considerable anger at her situation and at not being understood, even by those closest to her. The spiritual issue she is evidencing is a feeling of insecurity and lack of trust in life, in family, in herself. Telling were the last words "I just don't feel right," as if something is wrong and yet it cannot be named, captured and laid to rest. Lois's world is quaking beneath her. Insecure, without a sense of control, Lois became angry. Another experiencing a similar dynamic might become overwhelmed with fear. It is worth noting how in the verbatim Lois opened the visit, not the rabbi. She took charge. The need for control was vital for her. In this visit she quickly claimed it. In her life, it was more elusive.

How might the caregiver intervene meaningfully with a person whose major spiritual concern is to feel more secure in a life gone awry? To pretend the situation is not as frightening does not allay fears. It only engenders more reaction. Surely, Lois's family tried that approach and the results only served to enhance her anger. What might surprise us is that the best approach to help another cope with the fear and/or anger rooted in a sense of loss of control is to help the other name very specifically that of which they are most afraid. In identifying, specifying and claiming what is most awful to imagine, the suffering have overcome their subordination to the fear, the sense of being out of control. Indeed, in talking about what most intimidates him/her, the person suffering has regained control, if not of the situation, more importantly of his/herself. The suffering once again become the masters of their ship even as it is wind-tossed in the storm. In naming and claiming the fear, the suffering come to realize the "I" that transcends the ravages of even the worst of circumstances and in that there is comfort. Precisely what the sufferer may be most afraid of doing is what he/she needs to do to redress the spiritual imbalance caused by the insecurity of his/her predicament.

Let me share another Hassidic story from *Souls on Fire* that illustrates the point:

> Before his death, Rebbe Wolf told his servant, "I can see…A day will come, and it fills me with fear. The world will lose its stability and man his reason…A day will come and it makes me tremble. Do you hear me?"
>
> "Yes, Rebbe. I hear you."
>
> "I ask of you to tell it to our people. Tell them that on that day no one will be spared, not even men like me or you. We shall have to delve deep into our consciousness to find the spark. Will you tell them?"
>
> "Yes Rebbe. But…when that day comes what must they do in order not to go under? Do you know the remedy Rebbe?"
>
> The sick man sighed: "When that day comes, tell our people that I have foreseen it." He turned against the wall and was gone.[2]

What was the Rebbe's answer to his servant? What did "I have foreseen it" have to do with the servant's yearning for a remedy. In fact "I have foreseen it" was the remedy. When the world feels chaotic and out of control, when we are overcome by fear, having another tell us that they have seen our situation, that it could be seen, and contained, is itself a great gift. Think about it. When we have undergone a trauma in our life what is most hard is to visualize

2. Elie Wiesel, *Souls on Fire* (Vintage Books, 1973) p 88

it again. The scene is often too frightening for us to witness in our mind's eye. Yet precisely when we are able to see it again, when we find the courage to re-image the event we dread, we finally can be free of the terror it imposes on our life. It is the caregiver's work to make it safe enough for the one suffering to brave expressing the things they are most afraid will happen in their story of illness and loss. Rather than falsely attempt to protect the suffering, providing loving care means risking exploring the cave to help the sufferer identify all it contains. That won't make the darkness go away. But it will make the cave dweller more able to live and function in the darkness.

The Need to Belong

We all require community. Estrangement is at the foundation of all existential suffering, even as we discussed in great detail in Chapter Two. To live in this world and face the reality of our alone-ness, we need to belong. The community necessary for our spiritual well-being must offer us a sense of being understood and accepted for who we are, not on the basis of superficial presentation of ourselves, but in the deepest appreciation of our integrated reality. Most communities to which we belong fulfill our spiritual needs only partially at best. To the extent we hold back dimensions of our personality and story to the group, any acceptance we receive is compromised. We belong to many groups/communities. They include family, religious body, social organizations, political party, company of employment, just to name a few. Each may know only a portion of the self we are, and only in combination do we get the sense of membership we require to mitigate our aloneness.

The sick and suffering will frequently feel their sense of be-longing is affected severely by their illness. In its simplest form, the malady all too often prevents their participation in group life thereby making belonging more a matter of record than a living reality. At a deeper level, belonging is compromised because of the changed status within the sufferers. They no longer feel them-selves to be the same persons as once presented to the groups. They are less able, more dependent, more vulnerable. Are they still members in this eclipsed condition? At times, it is not just the onset of an acute situation that prompts the sense of alienation but a lifelong struggle with chronic problems, often veiled from others, that leaves a person feeling painfully disconnected. Let me share a verbatim account of a visit that reflects the struggle for belonging as it expresses itself in a lifetime of alienation made more painful in a time of heightened self-awareness.

Sara was a thirty-six-year-old single woman who at the time of this visit had her fifth operation for issues stemming from her lifelong struggle with Crone's Disease. The rabbi visiting was her congregational rabbi. Present at the time of the visit was her father and mother, both from out of town.

C1: Sara, do you mind if I sit down next to you?
P1: Sure, make yourself comfy.

C2: How did your operation go?
P2: This is my fifth one, rabbi, and it went just like the others went. They fixed whatever and I am waiting for the next one.

C3: Are you going to have another operation immediately?
P3: In Crone's Disease there is always another operation. No cure, just pain, operation, and more pain, and then waiting for the next one.

C4: That must be very frustrating and debilitating for you.
P4: Hey…them's the breaks…shit happens. Right rabbi?

C5: But at least you have a support system helping and rooting for you.
P5: My family has always been there for me. I have had this since I was fourteen, and they have been there no matter what.

C6: And all these flowers and cards. You must be a very popular person.

M1: She has an extremely good job, rabbi....My daughter is the head of a computer department for a large financial firm....These things come from the bosses and co-workers. They love her.

F1: Yeah, she's married to her job instead of to some nice guy.

P6: No men like to hear screams in the middle of the night, rabbi. Trust me, I know. A man can take a Crone's episode once, maybe twice, but then it's no calls.

C7: You are a bright and beautiful woman. I am sure there will be someone who will have the staying power.

M2: Find him rabbi, and my husband will put a new wing on your shul.

F2: If you find him, she won't have time. You see her job comes first.

P7: When you've hit enough brick walls in the man department, computers seem very tame.

C8: Not for me. My computer seems to have a mind of its own....But at least you have all these friends.

P8: Not friends, rabbi, acquaintances. They don't like the messy stuff that Crone's is made of. But I realize that and I don't blame them. (A technician enters and wants to take blood and urine samples.)

C9: Sara, do you mind if I say a prayer for your now?

P9: Sure, rabbi, whatever turns you on.

C10: (After the formal *mishebairach* the rabbi contin-ued) O God who protected our ancestors guide Sara in her journey. She has a terrible disease so please be kind to her. Give her the strength to cope and lessen her pain. Bring to her people who will care about her and will give her sup-port and friendship so she can get over the agonizing mo-ments with dignity and realize that some souls understand. Give wisdom to those who help in her care and give Sara patience to cope with the rest of us. Give her a whole heal-ing. Amen.

P10: (Sara has tears in her eyes) Rabbi, you have no idea what that meant to me. Thanks.

C11: I'll be back.
P11: I hope I'm not here.

In this visit Sara reflects the spiritual issue of needing to belong in powerful expression. She can find neither mate nor friend. No one truly accepts her in forging community. Even her parents, while present, demonstrate a certain detachment, as if Sara's life is too difficult for them to fathom. They are physically present but emotionally detached. The rabbi succeeds in building community with Sara in the here and now. He does so not so much through his words of support and encouragement in the visit. Rather he achieves communion with Sara in his prayer. Sara feels understood by the rabbi. His words reflect her story, and she feels an empathic bond. In that moment she is not alone. It models the hope for Sara more than all the rabbi's earlier words. Not surprising, at the close of the visit Sara expresses not the fatalism of earlier, but the hope for the future, all because community was forged by the rabbi entering deeply into Sara's world as a true friend.

The classic story in Hassidic literature reflecting on both the need for community and on how that community is achieved is told by Rebbe Nachman of Bratzlov. He related the story of a prince who went mad and thought himself a frog. The prince removed his clothes, got under the table, and ate only those foods appropriate to frogs. The King, beside himself with grief, offered a great reward to anyone who could cure his son. Many tried, none succeeded. Finally an unknown villager undertook the task. He began by removing his own clothes and getting down under the table with the prince. The surprised prince asked what he was doing there. The man replied, "I am a frog and this is where I belong." They continued to live together under the table for many days. Then one day the man put on his shirt. The prince asked, "What are you doing? Frogs don't wear shirts!" "True," replied the man, "but will wearing a shirt make me any less of a frog?" Wanting to connect with his friend, the prince too put on a shirt. Gradually, bit by bit, in similar fashion, the man took on all the behaviors of a man and the prince did likewise until the prince was conducting himself as befitted his rank and responsibility.

The caregiver in responding to the one who feels alone and different, like the prince in the above story, needs to get down and forge community. It was never clear in Rebbe Nachman's tale whether the prince, though functioning like a human, thought of himself still a frog. In the end, that does not matter. What does matter was that the prince had a sense of belonging to a community with the villager with whom he identified, which allowed him to live and function in meeting his life's responsibilities. No advice, no teaching, no kindness will substitute for joining the other in his/her world when the spiritual longing is for a sense of belonging. Of all the spiritual issues, this can be the most difficult for the caregiver to address. The caregiver must leave his/her world, at least for a while, in order to enter the world, no matter how bizarre, of the suffering other.

In unpacking the four core spiritual issues, we not only see that suffering has different dimensions. We also discover that to be a caregiver we need to play differing roles at the bedside to best respond to the issue most pressing. When a person is in need of affirmation, that is, to feel that he/she is OK in his/her diminished state of function, the role of the caregiver is to engage the suffering other as a loving parent, accepting the person suffering as whole with his/her infirmity. The work is one of listening, validating, without judgment or distance. When a person feels most acutely the spiritual need for value, the caregiver must allow him/herself to receive and/or collaborate with the suffering. Perhaps the caregiver will find a way to have the suffering teach him/her. The caregiver must be the receiver in this visit to afford a chance for the suffering to feel valuable in the here and now. If the sufferer is struggling to feel secure, the caregiver might take his/her cue from the role of coach, one who helps the other to find his/her inner courage to name the fears and take a sense of control even in a time when all seems so uncertain. Finally, when aloneness and the need to belong is the most pressing spiritual issue, the caregiver must, like the villager in Rebbe Nachman's story, become a friend, join with the other to build community.

A caregiver, whether he/she engages the work as rabbi, chaplain, or friend, cannot simply claim "My style of caregiving is…" Caregiving is not one-dimensional. It is not a style that needs to be claimed and perfected. On the contrary, to address the sufferer's spiritual issues at any given time, the caregiver has to constantly adapt his/her style to become the person the other needs to meet. If the caregiver enters every room with every patient in the same manner, the caregiver has missed his/her call. In truth this should really be no surprise. We are called to the *mitzvah* of caregiving out of the challenge of *imitatio Dei*, following in God's way. Yet look at what tradition says about the presence of the Divine.

"'I am the Lord your God.' It was necessary to make clear. Since the Holy One Blessed Be He appeared to them at the sea like a warrior in combat, and He appeared to them at Sinai like a scribe teaching Torah, and He appeared to them in Solomon's time like a young man, and He appeared to them in Daniel's time like an old man full of compassion…"[3]

God appeared to God's people making different impressions in accordance with their needs and circumstance. The caregiver in following in God's ways needs to do similarly. The love of God the

---

3. Tanchuma, Yitro

sick and suffering need to experience will show up differently in response to the spiritual struggle with which they are dealing. The figure below captures the thrust of what we have explicated in our discussion of spiritual assessment.

Spiritual Need	God's Presence	Pastoral Initiative	Pastoral Outcome
Affirmation	Parent	Acceptance	Loved
Value	Partner /Collaborator	Receiving /Learning	Meaning
Security	Coach	Encouragement /Challenge	Hope
Belonging	Friend	Sharing	Community

In order to do good caregiving, we must assess the spiritual issue. Then we must devise a way of engagement appropriate to best respond to that issue. Thirdly, we must utilize interventions specifically effective with the issues identified. Finally, we look for outcomes to confirm the effectiveness of our efforts and the correctness of our assessment. If the outcomes are not present, either we have made a wrong diagnosis as to the major spiritual issue present or our interventions were not on target.

Chapter 7
Healing Prayer

"Pray for me," a Hasid begged Rebbe Menachem-Mendl of Kotzk. "Things are going badly. I need your help; intercede on my behalf."

The Rebbe answered him harshly: "Are you too sick to say your own prayers?"

"I don't know how," responded the Hasid.

"What? You don't know how? That is your true problem!"

While we may never know the reasons for a specific illness and/or loss, Judaism has long taught that what happens to us is ordained by Divine decree. Divine providence is not only operational in human affairs, it is personal. Our fate is in response to our circumstance. All of life is therefore purposive. The Torah made clear that the suffering experienced by the people of Israel is designed to foster their return from their waywardness. "When you are persecuted and all these events will happen to you, then you will return to the Lord your God and hearken to His voice."[1] What is true for the people as a whole is true for each person as well in his/her own life's journey. Suffering is meant to refine us and help us reconnect to a spirituality often lost in the pursuit of the necessities and pleasures of the material world. The prayer of the sick is not only a means to an end, that of getting well again. The prayer of the sick is an end itself. Through illness, it is anticipated that the sick will turn with renewed vigor to

---

1. Deuteronomy 4:30

God, renew their spiritual life and in a new way, and repent.

I know reading the words of the last paragraph can engender strong feelings of resentment. Too often those who are healthy lord over the sick making judgments even as did the friends of Job. I do not mean in any way to support the judgmentalism that the well often use to engage the suffering. It is not possible to determine a person's degree of goodness on the basis of his/her life's circumstances. Long ago the prophets of Israel denounced the classicism by which those who had more treated those with less as inferior. What Judaism does however teach is that nothing in life occurs without meaning. While we do not know why someone does in fact suffer, we nevertheless need to see suffering as purposive, to learn from our story, rather than languish in a sense of victimization. Yes, the righteous get sick just as the wicked. We do not presume to know why. And yet we are still called upon to make use of our suffering story as a vehicle to move us closer to God, purify our being, and become the more spiritual selves we are capable of. Does that justify the suffering? We each have our own responses. At times I have my own doubts. It surely does not explain why we suffer when we look at the suffering of children, the elderly, those who are mentally ill and cannot change, to name a few obvious circumstances. Nonetheless, even though we cannot explain why we suffer, we are called upon to use suffering for self-renewal and refinement. All of our life's experience, its triumphs and defeats, its joys and griefs are meant to be lived so that they can help to shape us more truly in the form for which we were designed.

In truth, however, the sick and bereft are often blocked from the very access to the spiritual their circumstances are meant to engender. Caught up in the heaviness of their plight, consumed by worry and lament, they feel too detached from God to seek God. They are locked in the prison of their own ordeal. Even as we discussed in Chapter Three, God, while present, can only be accessed through the witnessing of the visitor. Like the Hasid in the story above, the sick and suffering oftentimes lose the words, the passion, the sense of relationship needed to pray.

The visitor, be he/she rabbi or friend, has the unique power and responsibility to open the passageway to the Divine for the sick and suffering. He/she has the wherewithal not only to reveal the presence of the holy at the bedside, as we discussed in detail in Chapter Five. He/she can bring the mute to expression, open up the channels of the soul that will serve to link the suffering to God. The transformative vehicle at the visitor's discretion is prayer.

The Shulchan Aruch in discussing the laws of *bikur cholim* makes it imperative for the visitor to pray for the sick to fulfill the *mitzvah*.[2] A careful reading of the text confirms that the prayer imperative refers to prayer at the bedside, in the presence of the sick, not prayer at the synagogue typically performed through the public recitation of the *mishebairach* (liturgical prayer for the sick). The Talmud taught that prayer for the sick in their presence can be recited in any language and be effective. It does not require Hebrew, the holy tongue, since the *Shekhina* is immediately present at the bed of the sick and the channel to the Divine is open.[3]

That said, it is surprising how uncommon it is for rabbis visiting the sick to recite a prayer for them at their bedside. My experience over the years with clergy of other faiths has shown that Christian and Muslim clerics are quick, at times perhaps too quick, to offer prayers in their visits. In fact, my priest and reverend students will often echo our sources unknowingly and say that a visit has not been a "visit" if no prayer was recited. Rabbis are more likely to tell a joke in a visit than recite a prayer. They tend to avoid God-talk in general. While at times a Torah lesson might be imparted to the sick, it is most unusual for the sick to be invited to speak of their personal spiritual struggle. The rabbi and for that matter other visitors seem to catch the absence of the holy in the sick person's experience rather than encounter the *Shekhina* inhering in the room.

So how can we learn to pray at the bedside? Christian clergy bring their prayers with them. There is something inauthentic in that. They, like many rabbis, don't experience the person in the bed as particularly inclined to a relationship with God, so they,

---

2. Shulchan Aruch, Yoreh Deah 335:4

3. TB Nedarim 40a

unlike rabbis, invoke God and create a prayerful moment. My sense is that rabbis are appropriately unwilling to bring to another that which does not feel like it belongs. To bring prayer where it is not invited is discourteous to both God and the worshipper. No, prayer cannot be brought into the room from without and be authentic. Prayer must emerge out of the sacred shared moment, the I-Thou encounter between the rabbi and the person suffering. When the rabbi and the one receiving care have had the intimacy born out of an expression of the inner hopes, fears, frustrations, and losses so close to the heart, prayer will feel like a natural response. More than be obligated to pray, they will feel a need to pray. Together they will feel impelled to invite God to sanctify the depth of their experience and bless the desires of their purest selves.

The Talmud already warned us, relative to our responsibility to pray thrice daily, that "if one's prayers are as by rote they will not be efficacious."[4] The three occasions each day when a Jew is responsible to pray conform to morning, afternoon, and night, when the changes of the natural world, the sun's rise, its setting and the eclipse of light into darkness are causes to stir the inner soul and prime the desire to express oneself to God. Prayer was meant not for God, but for humans, so they could have outlet for their spiritual excitation. From the earliest story of humankind as told in the Torah prayer was a spontaneous response to one's circumstances from triumph to despair. Visiting the sick, attending to the suffering needs to engender the desire for prayer, stimulate our spiritual consciousness so that rather than we recite the prayer, the prayer recites us. Our prayer needs to carry our soulful yearnings on its sound waves. The words are not questions but answers. We are revived in their annunciation.

In the most profound way when we pray with the suffering we are indeed praying with them, not for them. The prayer experience needs to be a shared one. As we have listened to the illness story or the story of loss we have become connected, our fates joined. After all it is a basic teaching that all Israel is essentially one and we are mutually responsible for each other.

---

4. Brachot 28b

The sick and suffering and the physically well are in essence just different parts of the same form. When the leg is wounded the arm feels it too, not out of sympathy, but because of the essential unity of the body. The relationship between the caregiver and the one cared for needs to happen out of that mindset. It is not "Here but for the grace of God go I" that serves as the operational dynamic. But "Here we are." The suffering person, however, is often too encumbered by his/her circumstance to pray. He/she frequently feels so consumed by his/her worries and fears that they are muted. It becomes the visitor's challenge to lead the way to God and to healing in drawing on the relationship to the Divine. It is the arm that may put the salve on the wounded leg inasmuch as the leg cannot tend to itself. At one with the suffering, yet detached enough emotionally to recognize that the story is of me but not me, the caregiver can serve as the resource to bring the needed yet previously inaccessible hope and renewal.

At times the hesitancy of the visitor to pray with the sick may emerge precisely from having achieved the intimacy that the *ben gil* relationship calls for. The visitor, be he/she rabbi or other, feels so close that inviting the suffering one to a prayerful moment seems a betrayal of the friend in becoming instead an authority. To ask, sometime in the visit, if the sick and suffering wants to pray is to assume the role of healer. It does indeed say, "I have a gift for us that you may not know is ours to partake of." It calls for the visitor to become the agent to access the holy, a one-up position vis-à-vis the infirmed other. To say the *barchu* in the midst of a congregation is to lead. Leadership at the bedside in calling for prayer is a transition from the listening/responding mode, so much the work of caregiving.

This is precisely the complex dynamic of the relationship between the suffering and those who care for them. At one level, the caregiver is meant to achieve a unity, a one-ness, born out of the purity of empathy. At another, the caregiver, as in our earlier paradigm, remains the arm, not the wounded leg, and must serve as leader to offer the treatment necessary for healing. The leadership, however, is not a leadership as in doing something for the other, but rather in doing something for ourselves. The leadership must always be preceded by a profound identification through which it is clear that any initiative suggested by the leader emerges not from a condescending perspective but out of a common yearning to be delivered from the awesome struggle shared.

Let us turn now to discuss more specifically the content and protocol for prayer. As we already underscored, the prayer expressed at the bedside needs to validate the realities of the situation as experienced by the suffering. It is not the truth of the predicament of the wounded other that is most telling in the content of a prayer but the wounded other's sense of his/her truth. When a sick man with cancer that has metastasized throughout his body and is at the terminal stages of his life asks us to pray for recovery, we need to hear it as the essential yearning for life. No matter that it would take a miracle for such a recovery to occur. No matter that as Jews, in accordance with tradition, we are not to pray for miracles.[5] We recite the prayer acknowledging the man's yearnings. We might say, "Dear God, Joe wants so much to live. Even with all the damage his disease has done, Joe wants to recover. He pleads with you to make a miracle on his behalf…" Through prayer we validate Joe's desire for life as a holy aspiration. We might name why he wants so much to live, what gives his life its meaning. In Joe's case, we as caregivers might correctly wish to avoid engendering false hope. We must be true to ourselves, in not pretending the reality is different from the medical diagnosis. The prayer we recite might continue, "If it is possible, Dear God, bring for Joe the deliverance he seeks. In all cases help him to know You are with him and he need not feel alone and afraid." I say "alone and afraid" if I have sensed that it is a part of the reason Joe is so invested in holding on to unrealistic hope. The words might be different if, say, Joe was concerned for his six-year-old daughter being without a Dad. Then I might say, "In all cases help Joe to know that his daughter Rachel will be protected by Your love and compassion."

The core truth here is that the prayer needs to honor the deepest yearnings, fears, hopes, dreams of the one in the bed. The

---

5. TB Brachot 54a

Talmud in discussing the *mitzvah* of *bikur cholim* makes the observation in the name of Rabbi Dimi: "Anyone who visits the sick causes them to live. While anyone who fails to visit the sick causes them to die."[6] The Talmud is perplexed by the quote and goes on to process its meaning, ultimately rewording the statement to say "Anyone who visits the sick can pray for their recovery. While anyone who doesn't visit cannot utter a prayer either for their recovery or their demise."

Rabbeinu Nissim, the primary medieval commentator on the tractate of Nedarim, explains the Talmudic passage as follows: "... There are many times when a person needs to pray for the sick person to expire, as in cases when the person ill is suffering greatly and it is impossible for him to recover....Therefore it [the Talmud] stated that one who visits the sick can at best be effective in prayer for the person to recover. However one who does not visit not only cannot be effective in prayer for the sick to recover (since s/he does not know the circumstance), but even to be effective in prayer for the sick person's demise he cannot (since he knows not what the sick person needs)."[7]

The prayer for someone to die is not a liturgical one. We would not be able to find it in a siddur. To recite a prayer reflective of the unique circumstances of another we must be creative in using the language and the metaphors that emerge from deep places within us. At times we may choose to share a chapter of Psalms. We may read it at the bedside to engender comfort and a sense of the holy in the midst of illnesses bleakness. What is important is that the Psalm not be presented without regard to the circumstances of the sick and his/her emotional struggle.

Choosing the right Psalm is both a skill and an art. We need to know the Psalms well enough to feel their relevance to different situations. We need to have an intuition about the suffering other to sense he/she will resonate with the words of the Psalmist, and feel them as his/her own.

What is most important to realize is that every feeling true to

---

6. Nedarim 40a

7. Ibid

the illness story of the suffering has a place in prayer and can be brought to God. Sometimes we may encounter a person overwhelmed with anger and the sense God has betrayed him/her. In his/her anger, he/she does not know how to be with God. The spiritual aloneness then becomes magnified. We need to be conduits between the angry sufferer and the Divine, not by chastising the sick one for his/her angry feelings nor by minimizing them. We need to bring the anger to God in prayer. Our prayer might sound something like this: "Dear God, Robyn is very angry with You this day. She had loved You her whole life and now when she needs You most she feels abandoned by You. Reveal yourself to her O God. Do not hide Your face from her…"

It would be wrong to deny another's truth in our prayer. Often I hear a chaplain begin prayer with "God, we thank You…" when thanks is hardly the feeling of the moment for the one suffering and afraid. We must believe for ourselves that God wants us in relationship with God, and that all true relationships have ups and downs, feelings of gratitude and at times anger. If the Psalms make anything clear it is that all feelings need to be shared with the Divine, even those that offer complaint, disappointment, and anger.

The great gift that we offer in joining with the suffering in prayer is that we honor their experiences as sacred and deserving of the attention of the Divine. Illness and loss in their most pernicious manifestation rob the one enduring them of the feelings that his/her experience is significant. The suffering tend to minimize their sad circumstances as the "junk" of their lives, something to be gotten over, a bad accident, in some profound ways almost shameful. Frequently the suffering do not complain of their situation because they do not deem it worthy of attention. Oppressed by their condition, they have not even the release of feeling the hero in their struggle. Instead they feel like actors in a badly written scene in which they are compelled to play. When prayer is expressed the sick and suffering experience a redemption more profound than we may at first realize. Their story is now not "junk" but holy. Their struggle is not a bad accident but heroic. The sick and suffering feel a renewed sense of pride. They are more able to live their suffering story, endure it as an important chapter of their lives. The shame, often an accompaniment of illness and loss, is transformed into meaning. Their experience through prayer becomes a saga, worthy of liturgy, as evidenced by the one who makes of their circumstance a prayer at the bedside.

In that regard, it does not really matter whether the one prayed for is a believer or not. The one offering the prayer and the one answering "amen" can come from wholly different religious traditions. When my wife and I had a child, the first and only for her, a girl after years of wondering if she might ever be a mother, one of her students in a pastoral care residency program came to visit. To our surprise, Yusef, an African-American Muslim chaplain, asked if he could say a prayer. My wife and I looked at each other. We had not felt prayerful at that moment, but we did not want to refuse. The Imam's spontaneous prayer for my wife, for the baby, for our family touched us deeply. It expressed the sacredness of our journey in a way we had not been able to access. In living the story, we had lost the perspective of its power. Yusef's simple prayer helped us to know what we already knew but lost touch with. Through his prayer our private struggle became a saga worthy of reverence. We cannot expect the patient to ask for prayer. As the Talmud teaches, "The prisoner cannot release himself from the jail."[8] The prisoner needs another. It is incumbent on the rabbi or visiting other to risk inviting prayer so that the suffering can discover and become conscious of the spirituality alive in him/herself and his/her story.

It is not prayer alone that can serve to help a person feel validated in his/her struggle. At times it can be enormously helpful if we can identify a scriptural story or passage that captures a theme similar to the one being lived out by the suffering. When we can point out to the person overwhelmed with the loss of a child that his/her story in some way parallels that of our father Jacob, who never did get over the assumed death of Joseph; when we can validate another's fear, despite his/her faith, by showing how Jacob was afraid, though he too had faith, when he had to confront his brother

---

8. Brachot 5b

Esau; when we can honor a person's confusion with the Divine when we reference Moses' struggle to comprehend the evil God was allowing to befall Israel in Egypt, we help the sufferer feel his/her story is holy, too, worthy of the literature of the sacred. Moreover, we help him/her to accept his/her feelings as "kosher" since even the giants of the faith have experienced them. Using Biblical imagery to help another find validation of his/her struggle needs to be done not as a sermon or didactic. Rather the Biblical image needs to be offered as a gentle invitation to identification that the suffering may choose to embrace or not. It must never be shared as our definitive interpretation. We might say to the suffering other that his/her situation recalls for us a Biblical encounter. And if he/she expresses interest, we might share it, and ask if it felt true for him/her. The sufferer may say yes in some ways, no in others. Then we can make use of the Biblical story to help further unpack the suffering one's experience in its subtleties and nuances.

I have visited with my students many times when they have offered prayers for patients and loved ones. As you might expect, the chaplain when offering the prayer will typically close his/her eyes. Since I was an observer I would often watch the patient. In many cases the patient rather than close his/her eyes actually had his/her eyes wide open. Frequently he/she during the prayer was gazing at the praying chaplain with adoration and love. It was as though the chaplain had given the patient a gift beyond the words. The chaplain made the patient's story holy, worthy of prayer. The gratitude expressed by the suffering one and evidenced in his/her eyes is profound and compelling. No gift to the caregiver could be more meaningful.

Let me close this chapter by sharing some helpful hints about prayer. It is a good idea in most circumstances when inviting the person visited into prayer to say, "What shall we pray for?" This way the sick and/or suffering can articulate and claim their need. They become empowered as we do their bidding. We do not want to pray *for* but rather we want to pray *with*. Use "we" rather than "he" or "she" as the language of request. Prayers are usually more effective when they are shorter, to the point, and directly capture the needs of the suffering. We must be bold enough to say what the sick and/or suffering may struggle to express. Thereby we help them to own their story and claim their oftentimes difficult realities. Name names. If the sick and/or suffering are concerned about children, make it personal by using their names. The same goes for the name of a spouse, parent, and so on. Don't always wait for the end of a visit to pray. At times prayer belongs in the middle or even at the opening of a visit. Don't run after the prayer. Sit, wait. Perhaps the feelings the prayer raised need to be processed, the tears talked about. Some of the most meaningful moments of intimacy occur after a prayer has been recited.

Oftentimes I am asked, "What is the difference between a chaplain's visit and the visit of a social worker or other mental health professional? What makes the spiritual visit unique?" Usually when this is asked it comes after the pastoral visit has been described for its therapeutic quality. In posing the question the one asking is trying to discern "where is God in all of this listening and presence that has been described."

From my perspective, pastoral care may be done by a nurse, a physician, a social worker or even a maintenance person. It is not who does it that defines its reality but the kind of care being given. If the care offered helps the patient feel the presence of the "holy" or transcendent in the midst of his/her struggle, if the patient through the encounter finds meaning in the maelstrom of his/her circumstance, it was indeed a pastoral visit whatever else it also may have been and no matter who performed it.

Prayer and the invocation of the Divine is an affirmation of the spirituality now alive for the patient and his/her visitors. The prayer belongs to both and neither has to be ordained to make it appropriate. The question as to what constitutes pastoral care is answered in the "meeting" that occurs between two persons in the authentic moment. Unlike caring in other forms, pastoral care is transactional, that is, in the process of caring both the recipient and the one providing care are changed. Both feel the intimacy born out of the we-ness established. While no change may have occurred relative to the external circumstances of the sufferer, something profound has happened, each has transcended his/her limitations by joining the other. The new creation is indeed a gift and impels prayer. The pastoral visit is a blessed moment in what feels for many an accursed time. Through prayer that blessed moment becomes not a distraction but indeed the core reality, a connection to the infinite that offers hope in the depth of finitude.

Chapter 8
Waiting on Shame

As a teen, Elie Wiesel went to a Nazi labor camp with the father he loved – they struggled there, father and son to survive. He cared for his father, even in the context of great deprevation. Yet as much as he loved his father, that was not the only feeling he felt in those trying times.

In his classic *Night*, Wiesel tells the story that once, after a long march, he could not find his father and he found surprising and unbidden feelings arise within himself.

> *Don't let me find him. If only I could get rid of this dead weight, so that I could use all my strength to struggle for my own survival, and only worry about myself.*
>
> *Immediately I felt ashamed of myself, ashamed forever.*[1]

The above account parallels the inner dynamics of many family members in the wake of their loved one's prolonged illness and debilitation. Yes, family members love their sick relative. Yes, they want for him/her to recover. Yes, they will spare no effort to bring comfort and relief. But other feelings are often also present, feelings less attractive and unbidden. Truth be told, Wiesel's emotions are not the feelings of a derelict son. Nothing is more clear than Wiesel's love for his father. That did not prevent him from experiencing the

---

1. Elie Wiesel, *Night*, p118

paradoxical feelings of being overwhelmed with the burden of worry, responsibility and fear that he would fail in his role as a caring son to protect his father or that his success in saving him might come at the expense of his own survival. To love another, to care for them deeply, engenders many feelings, some that produce pride, others that cause us to feel ashamed.

In this chapter we will explore shame as an operating dynamic in our life and relationships. We will frame shame's presence in language both theological and psychological. We will discern how to recognize shame's presence in the work of caregiving and how to respond to it once revealed. Most importantly, we will normalize the presence of shame, so that we can attend to it in our efforts to help others, rather than ride over it unconsciously and often at great cost.

Shame has become a much talked about issue in our times. The theoretical literature around addiction, its causes and treatment, has zeroed in on shame as a prevailing dynamic. Importantly, we need to define shame and distinguish it from its closely associated cousin, guilt.

Shame has come to be understood in modern thought as an experience of inner diminishment often related to some external stimuli. To experience shame is to experience a sense of inner lacking, a failure to have lived up to one's own sense of what one should be. While shame may be triggered by an external event, say forgetting one's lines in a public speaking engagement, it is not the event itself that is the source of the sense of inadequacy associated with shame, but one's self-concept as a competent, capable, talented individual that may have gotten compromised in the experience.

Shame, as Helen Merrel Lynd points out in her seminal work on the topic *On Shame and the Search for Identity*, is forever self-involving.[2] In contradistinction to guilt, it is not about what one did but rather about who one is. In one's sense of guilt, the feeling is, "I made a mistake." In the experience of shame, one feels "I am

---

2. Helen Merrel Lynd, *On Shame and the Search for Identity* (New York, Science Editions, 1958) Chapter 2

a mistake." The experience of guilt involves the disappointment of the expectations of others, a parent, a tradition, a community. In shame, the one disappointed is the self. When encountering shame, we are painfully conscious that we are not who we believed we were supposed to be.

Precisely because shame is self-involving it is not easily healed. In response to the experience of having done something wrong, one can find many defenses to lighten the load. One can rationalize and explain the reasons for the mistake. One can lessen the consequences of the error, show that it all turned out fine in the end. One can apologize to the offended other and be forgiven. Shame knows no such relief. Because in shame one experiences oneself as the mistake; any effort at reinterpretation only further highlights his/her inadequacy. Since it is not about the other, forgiveness is irrelevant. And since shame is marginally related with the action itself, it is of no use to say it did not matter. Take our example of the speaker who forgot his/her lines. It does not matter that the speech was a success, that no "wrong" was committed, that the speaker was up all night and can excuse him/herself. If the speaker is experiencing shame, he/she feels severely wounded by his/her sense of being inadequate in comparison to his/her sense of who he/she should be. The failure is personal and not expungable.

The consequences of a sense of shame in some instances can be devastating. Let's look at a verbatim snippet from a visit made by one of my chaplain-interns some years ago, which illustrates the havoc a sense of shame can wreak in a person's life. Lucy was a forty-six-year-old unmarried Latina woman. She was hospitalized in the aftermath of a fall in her home. She had been hospitalized numerous times over the past ten years, all because of pain that would not subside. The physicians found Lucy's pain mystifying. They could detect no physiological symptoms that would explain it. At times, Lucy's frequent demand for pain medication was seen by the medical staff as an unhealthy dependency and suspicions of an addiction were raised. She was given placebos to see how much of her pain was the product of her mind alone. The medical staff treated Lucy with a disdain, born from a judgment that she was manipulating the system rather than striving to get well. The chaplain, also a Latino, and a man of similar age to Lucy, found Lucy to be open to visits but conversations tended to be for the most part circular and superficial. The visit recorded below was the chaplain's fifth with Lucy. Lucy was described as an attractive woman. Her room was graced by a vase of flowers, candies and cookies. Her right leg was bandaged to the ankle.

C1: Hello, Lucy. You look well today. You have lipstick on!

P1: Yes, I feel better. (Smiling)

C2: That makes me feel good. So tell me what's happening in your life?

P2: I was in pain earlier today (said with anger). They refused to give me my medication. I called the doctor and he told them to give me my medication because I have suffered enough.

C3: So the doctor took care of your medication.

P3: Yes, he was upset because they refused to give it to me when I wanted it (she pauses). My problems started all in 1985. I went shopping with my little boy Steven, and while we were looking in a dress shop, a car jumped the sidewalk and ran over me and my son. My son was then hit again and died instantly. Forgive me if I begin to cry.

C4: Cry all you want. It's a good thing to let out all that pain. I cry all the time.

P4: I'm on a hunger strike against the nurses on the floor.

C5: Why is that?

P5: On this floor the nurses have no compassion, except one, who always gives me my medication and doesn't let me suffer.

The visit continued with Lucy speaking of her anger at her treatment and the pain that never goes away.

In many ways the work of pastoral care, not unlike medical care, is that of a detective. One needs to look for the spiritual issues, sometimes obscured, in the same way the physician searches for the underlying medical problem. Lucy is languishing in her pain, her life held captive. The source needs to be considered in the context of her story. What is the oppressive truth, so overwhelming that Lucy cannot move on even if she does have some pain? The answer was revealed when Lucy confided to the chaplain the story of the death of her son Steven. Lucy's story is the story of a mother who lost a child. No, she did more than lose a child; she was there and unable to protect him. They were looking at dresses, not buying toys. In the service of her agenda, they both were in the place to be struck by a car, Steven being killed. What Lucy has experienced over the years since has been relentless and unmitigated shame, the shame of a mother who failed to protect her son. In her own sense of who she was meant to be she failed the ultimate failure. Lucy's pain is rooted in her deep and haunting disappointment in herself. Medication helps her to forget; that is the only relief she knows. Unlike guilt, which can be rationalized, externalized, cleansed, shame is internal and about who one is or is not. Does Lucy's self-diminishment make sense? Not really. She could hardly be said to be at fault. But that reasoning will not help alleviate Lucy's shame any more than telling an adult he/she was not responsible for the sexual molestation endured as a child will make the shame disappear. Shame is not like guilt. It allows no argument, no matter how reasoned.

The story of child loss for mothers is often about shame. In my own experience in the rabbinate, I have seen numerous mothers become in many important ways "dead" to the world in the aftermath of the death of their child. Friends, family, even their own husbands do not understand what is happening to them. They may well perform routines but yet they remain somehow detached from life. Many novels and movie scripts have told the story of a mother who lapsed into alcoholism or debilitating depression after the death of their child. In the W. Somerset Maugham classic *The Razor's Edge*, the character Sophie loses herself entirely to drink and decadence because of her inability to tolerate the sense of her failure as a mother.[3] Friends, and in particular the story's hero, spare no effort to save her. Yet in the end it is all in vain. Similar to Lucy in our verbatim, the shame is too hot to be touched; as soon as it manifests itself, it quickly shifts to anger or it escapes in some other diversion.

The situations that engender shame are as numerous and diverse as the content of life itself. Some shame renders a bearer virtually incapacitated, as on occasions when parents have endured the death of a child, or perhaps where one has failed in a career or sustained the dissolution of a marriage. The blows to one's sense of who one ought to have been and did not realize as protective parent, competent professional or loving partner can be devastating. Some shame is less pernicious. Yet in all cases, the experience of shame tends to cause a constriction of the self. Typically, when we have felt shame, we pledge to ourselves never to be caught in that predicament again. Barbara Streisand once forgot her lyrics in a live performance. In response, for the next decade, she chose not to perform live concerts. Fear of shame causes us to lose our spontaneity, become more guarded and deliberate. We are less inclined to risk.

As caregivers, it is important to recognize that the illness story is often punctuated by experiences of shame. The man who has spent a career as a self-reliant powerful executive may well feel shame at his state of incapacity where he is dependent on the kindness of others. He feels himself an intolerable failure. He would rather die than give up his independence. No matter how many family members tell him that they need him, want him, love him and that he is no burden, it will not matter. It is not them that he fails in his present circumstance, but himself. It is his own image he cannot endure. The same holds true for the woman who feels robbed by her condition from the caregiving role she enjoyed as the family matriarch. It is not the disappointment of the others,

---

3. W. Somerset Maugham, *The Razor's Edge* (New York, Doubleday, 1944)

that they will not have the Thanksgiving dinner in her home, that is unbearable. She believes them when they tell her a restaurant will do fine. What she cannot bear is her disappointment in her self. She feels depleted of her self-esteem, forced to confront a self-image she does not recognize or find acceptable.

Family members often carry their own shame in the illness story. Frequently, they have ambivalent feelings in response to their loved one's circumstances. At one level, yes, they want their father or mother to recover, their husband or wife to come home. But they also struggle with the fear of lingering chronic illness. It is hard to see another in pain, especially one who is loved. They worry about the depletion of financial resources were the parent either to languish or experience a slow decline. They worry about their own strength to meet the challenges of providing care over a protracted period and a worsening of the disease state. Like Elie Wiesel in the vignette with which we began the chapter, one of the feelings present to most caregivers may be the hope their loved one will die and this horrible saga will come to an end. And yet that very feeling is so uncomfortable to acknowledge even to the privacy of one's own self that often it is avoided at all costs. To acknowledge the hope for the demise of the other would induce a powerful experience of shame. As we have discussed, the one relief we have from shame is forgetfulness. Often times the "busy-ness" we see in family members over functioning at the bedside of the one they love reflects not their unbounded devotion but rather should be seen as compensatory activity to mitigate the sense of shame they would otherwise have to face, the unbidden feelings of wanting to bring this story to an end.

When a caregiver, be he/she a chaplain, rabbi, or friend, enters the arena of the sick, he/she needs to be cautious of the assumptions made. Too often I hear the caregiver affirm the love of the family for the sick in idealized terms. He/she is frequently quick to bless the attending husband, wife, or children as devoted and heroic in the service of their loved one. Correspondingly he/she will remark to the one sick on how fortunate he/she is to have a family so committed to his/her care. What the caregiver has done in framing what he/she is experiencing in those terms is to capture only one side of a complex story. Sure love is present and commitment, too. But no family is without its complexity of dynamics. And in idealizing the relationship in purely positive terms the possibility of validating the ambivalence and yes the shameful desires of both the family and even of the sick themselves is negated. For in truth, the sick and dependent carry their own ambivalent feeling toward the ones caring for them. The are grateful for the gift of their loved ones' care. Yet like all who are dependent, they hate the persons they must rely on as much as they hate themselves for needing them.

So how do we respond to the shame so often present in the illness story? One thing is clear: We cannot relieve shame by talking through it as we might many of life's other issues. And we cannot relieve shame by simply helping the other to express the feeling. As we discussed earlier, shame does not lend itself to be rationalized away and because it is about the core sense of who one is, giving voice to it alone will not release it. In fact, directly talking to another about their shame will likely induce denial and/or anger. In response to shame, the caregiver needs to apply an entirely different way of responding. The way of loving another in their time of shame can be gleaned from sources very much found within our tradition. Let us explore a couple of Torah stories of shame.

In the Book of Numbers we are told of an incident in which Miriam and Aaron, Moses' sister and brother, spoke badly about Moses' questioning something in his domestic life described as "the Kushite woman which he took."[4] God, in the account, was angered by their talk against Moses. God called them both outside the camp and chastised them and challenged their assumption that they knew what was right to do just as well as Moses did. God criticized them for what in tradition is called *lashon harah*, evil speech about another. Miriam was left with leprosy as a consequence of her sin. As the story unfolds, Aaron is painfully aware of his sister's distress. He pleaded with Moses to pray for Miriam that she should be cured. Moses did indeed pray for Miriam. In response he was

---

4. Numbers 12:1

told by God, "If her father were to spit in her face would she not be ashamed for seven days? Let her remain outside the camp for seven days, then to return."[5]

The story is at first mystifying. Miriam was living with a disease. Moses prayed for her cure. We are not told whether in fact God relieved her of her disease or not. All we are told is that God said that she would need seven days outside the camp before returning. What's going on? The answer is that Miriam's hurt was in fact two-fold. At one level, of course, she was afflicted with a terrible malady needing cure. But she also suffered something far more pernicious. She experienced the shame of having been publicly censured by God for her evil talk and that against her own brother. The leprosy was not only a plague of its own. It was a sign of God's disappointment in her and indeed became a source of her own disappointment in herself. God's answer to Moses' prayer makes sense in this context. God said, as it were, to Moses, of course I can cure her of her disease but she suffers from an emotional/spiritual issue as well. She suffers from shame. God went on to explain the shame as if having been spit on by one's parent. God told Moses, "The disease I can cure, but the shame will require its own healing. It will take time. She will need to be outside the camp, living with her own sense of inadequacy."

How is Miriam's sense of shame healed? The Torah gives us an important conclusion to the drama. It tells us that indeed Miriam remained outside the camp for seven days, as God said would need to happen. It closes the story by telling us "the people did not travel until Miriam was restored to the camp."[6] Here lies the great truth. Inasmuch as shame is not about some external act but about the essence of who one is, the only way to bring about healing is to receive the other with their shame and affirm thereby their worth. Excusing the shame, avoiding the shame, minimizing the shame all only serve to keep the one enduring it stuck in shame's net. In accepting the person and their sense of shame for what it is, we say to the other, "Yes, you may feel lacking in your sense of who you

---

5. Numbers 12:14
6. Numbers 12:15

should be. You may feel inadequate. Yet with it all we want you to know you are loved and acceptable to us. Your sense of limitation does not make you any less good to us or any less deserving of community." Thus the response of the People of Israel to Miriam, a woman who they loved and admired, was not to pretend she was not compromised, nor to make excuses for her. All that would do would be to heighten the awareness that her shameful feelings are indeed significant and in need of remediation. Instead, what the people do is simply wait for Miriam, accept her as substantial and important even in her less than flattering time. In waiting, they affirm Miriam's intactness even when she feels herself inadequate. Her shame is not so much cured as it is made acceptable, telling her she is OK even when she does not feel OK. No, more, not telling her, but showing her in action, in the waiting, that she is OK, even when she does not feel OK.

Healing shame is not about treating an experience. As we have made clear, shame is about the self, not an event. To help another we need receive him/her with his/her shame. In my own life I can recall sharing with a therapist a shameful aspect of myself that I never shared with another. It took two years of trust-building for me to reveal my source of shame and I wept as I spoke it. In truth it was, I realized, something someone else might consider a small matter. For me it was a burden I could barely utter. The therapist listened and nodded. She did not focus on my source of shame. She focused on me. With tenderness, she showed me she understood how difficult it was for me to express my shame. Then she just accepted me not differently than before I spoke. It was as if I just shared any other information in my therapy, no less and no more. The session soon came to an end. My shame was spoken to another, and I was intact. I was now OK to another with my shame, and consequently in important ways more OK with myself as well.

In my supervision of students in Clinical Pastoral Education, sometimes shameful material comes up. I can remember one young woman who in the very emotional process of CPE came to own her experience of having been molested by her father. I did not invite her story, nor did I tend to it. Rather, when she shared it with me in her supervision hour, I simply affirmed her saying "You're OK" over and over as she spoke what she needed to say. The woman went on to explore her experience later in therapy. Yet she always claimed the gift I gave her of simply receiving her with her shame was the pivotal beginning of her healing journey. It was the waiting on shame, even as Israel waited on Miriam in the wilderness, that validated the other as worthy and good even in his/her sense of diminishment. Carl Jung observed of his patients that "the patient does not feel himself accepted unless the very worst in him is accepted too."[7]

As caregivers we need to engender the trust and warmth sufficient to help others feel they can risk voicing their shame. Moreover, we need to demonstrate that we have good boundaries so others will feel if they share their shame they will be respected rather than analyzed or taken care of. Much of assessment of good caregiving can be gleaned by observing what is said and not said in the room. Do we help families feel safe enough to acknowledge their ambivalence? Can we tolerate another's sense of inadequacy and receive him/her in the brokenness or do we rather quickly try to repair him/her? Do we get surprised in our visits with the unexpected revelation or are our conversations fairly predictable?

To be sure, shameful feelings are present in the stories of sickness and loss. At times they may evidence themselves in the prevailing silence between the family members and the ones they love. At times they can be seen in the constricted mannerisms of the one in the bed often erroneously diagnosed as depression. At times they may reveal themselves in the patient's or family's angry outbursts, prevailing moodiness, or avoidance of relational conversation. The role of the pastoral care visitor is to affect a respectful presence, one that will lead the one feeling shame to believe he/she can risk unburdening him/herself by sharing his/her sense of inadequacy and self-disappointment. Unlike much of what we discussed earlier in framing the pastoral role as becoming a *ben*

---

7. Carl G. Jung, *Modern Man in Search of a Soul* (New York, Harcourt Trade, 1955)

gil often by actually facilitating a sharing, when shame is the p-
vailing issue one must wait. At times the waiting is rewarded with
trust. At other times it is not. But one can be certain that if
shame is the dynamic most pressing, pastoral interventions other
than waiting will not be helpful. Instead, they will likely engender
rage and/or detachment. They will inflict more hurt than help,
often confusing the caregiver.

Let me close this chapter by exploring briefly the Biblical story
most recognizably dealing with shame. Again we go to the Garden,
again to visit the experience of Adam and Eve. The Torah makes
clear that the initial feeling Adam and Eve had to deal with after
the sin of eating the forbidden fruit was shame. Their first awareness was of their own nakedness. Their first impulse was to cover
themselves. Hiding both from each other and then from God is a
behavioral manifestation of shame. They were conscious for the
first time of their inadequacies. They were painfully aware that
they were flawed. It is not surprising then when God gave each the
opportunity to confess, take responsibility and be forgiven, they
chose instead to blame each other. They knew that no forgiveness from God would relieve their shame. They suffered from the
consciousness of who they were more than from the consequences
of what they did. Avoidance is the only relief and even that is
shallow. God meted out punishment to Adam and Eve. They
are never explicitly forgiven. Indeed since it is not the sin that
plagued them but their own failure to be worthy as God's handi-
craft, no forgiveness would matter. Yet God did in fact respond to
the shame. The last verse of that episode in the Torah reads: "And
the Lord God made clothes of skins for Adam and his wife and he
clothed them."[8] The poignancy of this passage must not be missed.
In response to shame, no words of forgiveness will bring relief. As
we have described, the issue of shame is who one is, not what one
did. The loving response to shame is expressed in receiving the
other with his/her inadequacy, accepting the other as worthy even
in his/her brokenness. In responding to shame we do not deny the
truth of the other's experiences of him/herself. We simply show

8. Genesis 3:21

by our actions that we love him/her anyway. God gave Adam and Eve the most loving possible response. God gave evidence of God's love for them, not only by making clothes for them in their sense of nakedness, but by dressing them. God, God's self became Adam and Eve's tailor, and yes, valet. In serving God's creations even in their broken state, God affirmed their value and meaning. They were loved with their shame. It does not make the shame go away. It does, however, help make the ones suffering more able to love themselves even as they have been loved.

Chapter 9
Separation and Attachment

In the end, the time comes for the infant to emerge into the world. Immediately that same angel comes and informs the infant, "It's time for you to enter the world."

The infant responds, "Why do you want to send me into the world?"

The angel says, "My child, know that you had no choice in your creation and now no choice about being born; no choice about your death, and no choice about giving an account for your life before the Holy One Blessed Be He."

The infant does not want to leave and has to be physically compelled. The candle above the infant's head is then extinguished. The infant is forcibly brought into the world. Immediately he/she forgets all he/she saw, all that was his/ her prior knowledge.

And why does the infant cry? For the lost place of comfort and peace. A whole world lost to him/her...[1]

All living from its very inception is about loss. In the language of the Medrash, the theme is reflected in the journey of the person from his/her heavenly home into this world of chaos and struggle. In the language of developmental psychology, it is reflected in the anxiety of the infant forced at birth to adjust to his/her new environment, separated from the safety and comfort of mother's womb. And birth is not an aberration. Rather it is reflective of the challenge of the human experience.

1. Tanchuma, Pikudei

Maturity is at its core about successfully negotiating separation, acknowledging loss. The Torah in early Genesis frames the gift of marital union with "Therefore a man will leave his father and mother and cleave to his wife..."[2] There can be no new union without a separation from the old. Personality theorists have long argued that mental health is rooted in the early life challenges of separating from maternal dependency. The child needs the supportive environment provided for the most part by good parenting for him/her to find the courage to become autonomous and individual, a healthy self. To be is to separate. To separate is to sustain losses. Let us spend some time reflecting on these essential truths from the vantage point of Jewish theology.

Jewish tradition understands the work of the human being in this world is to choose. In choosing good over evil, right over wrong, the spiritual over the material, we fulfill our mission and can return successfully to the home from which we were banished at birth. This world, unlike its spiritual counterpart, is finite. Choice is always either/or, never both/and. If I am choosing to be here I cannot at the same time be there. If I choose to do this, I cannot at the same time do that. Space and time are the constraints that limit all of us and force us to choose if we are to live. Saying "yes" to one thing means saying "no" to another, if not forever at least for now. It is precisely because making choices involves letting go that it produces so much anxiety. Erich Fromm wrote powerfully of the human being's struggle to choose in his classic *Escape from Freedom*. There he argued that to be free is not, in fact, to have the capacity to choose but rather to have the courage to be making choices.[3] Judaism expressed the challenge most compellingly in the Torah's call "And you shall choose life".[4] The evil inclination is often referred to in rabbinic literature as the "yeast within the dough," that which causes the dough to ferment by inactivity. The human condition is understood to be rooted naturally in the material and self-serving. Holiness is referred to as *kedushah*,

2. Genesis 2:24

3. Erich Fromm, *Escape from Freedom* (New York, Avon, 1965) p39ff

4. Deuteronomy 30:19

literally meaning separation. To sin is to fail to choose. To do an *avairah* literally is to "pass-over," to languish when given the opportunity to meaningfully separate. When the Torah challenged the Jew "*Kedoshim* (plural of *kadosh*) you shall be" it was placing on him/her the sacred work of separation.

With reference to good and evil, the Talmud makes a surprising observation. It teaches that the evil inclination, the *yetzer harah*, is with a person from birth, while the good inclination, the *yetzer tov*, does not emerge until the age of puberty.[5] The idea is at first counter-intuitive. Children often demonstrate what appears to be a holy innocence, while true wickedness seems reserved for adult behavior. The Talmud sees it otherwise. When children do "good" they are not choosing but mimicking the behavior deemed appropriate for adults. They have not reached a level of consciousness sufficient to be making choices. It is the evil inclination, the instinct, not true choice, that governs them. Only a conscious adult can choose, exercise the good inclination, and commit an act of *kedushah*, separation.

Separation, the pursuit of holiness, while the challenge of life does not come without a sense of loss. The fact that holiness is an act of separation means that it requires forsaking one dimension of the self to pursue the excellence of another. The Talmud makes the poignant comment that after death, at the time of the ultimate judgment, the righteous will look at their evil inclination, not acted upon, and they will cry.[6] Astounded by its size, they will wonder at their ability to have withstood its influence. Body and soul in Jewish tradition reflect the duality of earth and spirit comprising the human being. After death, the soul, now separated from the body, according to rabbinic sources, hovers around its former partner, the body, pained at the loss caused by the separation in death.[7] If the angel in the story with which we opened the chapter had to force the infant out of its heavenly home into the material world, it is only half the saga. That same angel, the Talmud teaches, calls

---

5. Avot D'Rabbi Natan 16:2

6. TB Succah 52b

7. Shulchan Aruch, Yoreh Deah 384.3

the person back, only this time he/she does not want to leave his/her earthly residence, and wants desperately to remain.

It is not only the individual's spiritual story that has as its central theme separation and loss. Humanity as a whole is in great measure living out the same drama on a greater stage. The Torah tells us that Adam and Eve were placed in the Garden of Eden with the task to work the Garden and guard it. The most significant consequence of their sin was banishment from the Garden, exile not only from their designated home but from their designated roles. Ever since, the human challenge has been to find the way back to the Garden, to reclaim that which was lost. Indeed, from the perspective of the theologian, humankind's great mistake has been in seeking the Garden by attempting to convert the ordinary into paradise rather than converting itself so that it might be worthy of return. Humanity has struggled to accept its loss, unable or unwilling to live the truth of its banishment, preferring instead the illusion that the Garden of Eden is but a pleasure-thrill away.

The story of the Jewish people parallels the human drama. In the prayer service we regularly recite "And because of our sins we were exiled from our land…" (*Musaf* liturgy). Israel's exile shapes her story of near two thousand years. It is a story of loss in most profound manifestations. Every persecution, every tragedy has been experienced in the context of the Exile. The Jewish people have understood that even as horrific a tragedy as the Holocaust needs to be remembered in the context of Tisha B'Av, and the loss of the national home and sovereignty. The challenge for Israel, not different from humanity as a whole, is to accept the loss for the core reality it represents. Only in embracing the truth of the loss, painful as that may be, can the possibility of return be realized and Israel's destiny be fulfilled.

This brings us to a critical addition to our discussion. Loss and separation are indeed the key elements to the story of persons, humanity and the Jewish people. But not loss and separation alone. Separation is but one half of the challenge of life. The other is attachment. In our finitude, we accept the loss associated with separation not for its own sake. We experience the full dynamic of separation because we know that it is the price we must pay to attach to something new and more necessary to us. Humanity must accept its post-Garden status with its attendant hurt in order to yet attach to the Garden restored. Israel must embrace the Exile with its attendant suffering so that it might return, and reattach to its land and rightful role. The individual in the context of his/her life must come to accept the loss of the pre-Garden unity with the holy so that he/she can prepare for a future reconciliation. In denying or avoiding the loss, we stay stuck in allegiance to that which we imagine to be. That leaves less room for attachment to our true destiny. In hanging on to pretense, we compromise that which is the promise and the hope.

The great truth of existence is that life is about separation and attachment. Failure to do the work of separation inevitably costs us dearly in limiting opportunities for the attachments we most need and desire.

I can remember the challenge faced by one of my students in CPE. Ruth was a Catholic sister, mature of years, who struggled in her relationship with the other sisters in her order of nuns. She came in her mid-sixties into CPE as the last hope to find a direction for her life in religious service. Ruth was earnest and hardworking. She visited patients with a resolve to care. But Ruth struggled to cultivate relationships with patients and for that matter with her peers in CPE and with me in supervision. She just seemed unable to become a friend to those who needed companionship. While wanting so much to be helpful she could neither respond to the aloneness of others nor find friendship for herself. The struggle of her life in her religious community was replayed in CPE. Exasperated with Ruth's block and not knowing how to intervene meaningfully, I listened to Ruth and waited. And then it came.

One day in supervision, I asked Ruth about the losses in her life. She told me in response that she had always struggled to acknowledge loss. She went on to explain that her struggle with loss had its source in her youth. When only a five-year-old, her father died. Her mother and the family decided to protect Ruth from the pain of her father's death. They hid the truth of his death from her. She was never told. To this day, Ruth told me, she had never grieved his passing even though she felt the overwhelming heaviness of his death. In the context of Ruth's story, her struggle with relationship became clear. Ruth had never grieved. She had not faced the awful loss of her childhood. Taught to fear loss as too terrible to endure, she would live life devoid of attachment. Her fear of loss caused her to flee any intimacy lest she have to face its termination. Despite the good intentions of her mother, the message she was given in her youth was that she could not survive the pain of separation. The only way she knew to live a life without the threat of that pain was to isolate. The work she needed to do as a caregiver was not that of attachment but rather that of separation. It was only in facing her losses and experiencing the concomitant hurt that she would find the courage to be vulnerable in living life in relationship. Ruth's story is more common than we might first imagine, at least in the dynamic if not in the detail. When we discover men and women who struggle with intimacy and/or commitment, most often the source is not in a resistance to deep relationship but in the fear and pain of separation intimacy puts them at risk for. Sometimes the loss that triggered that fear happened early in life and needs time to uncover. Sometimes the loss is more recent. How many a divorced or widowed man or woman decline opportunity for new love and happiness because they are fearful of the cost they might pay in pain suffered at the disappointment if the relationship failed or still worse the loss experienced should they love and lose again.

One of the greatest gifts of religion in general and of Judaism in particular is the support it offers for coping with loss. By giving us rituals of closure and grief, religion sets up for us structured pathways to help us express the hurt in our losses so we need not fear either pain's power or its potential for chaos. Judaism formalizes loss and mandates ritual practices at the time of death. The burial rituals force a recognition, painful though it may be, that the dead are indeed dead. Tradition disdains any cosmetic makeup of the deceased. It makes the act of burial itself, shoveling dirt on the coffin, a holy act, a *mitzvah* to be performed by family and loved ones. *Shiva* mandates crying and a withdrawal from the social fabric of everyday living. It makes the immediate family "mourners," for a week, and then to a lesser degree for a month, and for parents for as long as a year. No room for denial here, no escape from the impact of loss. And yet in entering the ritual one can let go and not be afraid. The grief has a context, boundaries, and behaviors. Moreover, the community supports the individual's process and accepts its role as a source to provide safety and comfort.

It is not in the most glaring experience of loss, the death of a loved one, alone that Judaism honors the work of facing loss in order to renew life. Jewish tradition calls upon its practitioners to validate many losses through ritual. The end of marriage through divorce requires a *Get*, a document of divorce. The *Get* is given by the husband to the wife in a religious ceremony with the words "You are hereby divorced from me and permitted to marry any man." No illusion here about what is happening. The separation is complete to make room for new attachments. When the Sabbath and Jewish Holidays come to a close, tradition mandates the recitation of *Havdalah*. Prayers and blessing are recited over wine, candle, and spice bringing closure to the holy so that we might again enter the secular weekday world. *Havdalah* means separation. Indeed separation in order to attach again. Part of the ceremony at the Sabbath's close is the inhaling of spices, to revive us and bring comfort in our time of sadness and loss. Completion of a tractate of the Talmud requires a *siyum*, a celebration of closure with attendant prayers of thanksgiving. In the liturgical prayers recited at the *siyum* is embedded the recognition that with the celebration comes a loss and a need to move on to begin new tractates for study.

Many of our life's losses, however, do not fall within the parameters of religious ritual and practice. They are frequently gradual losses that do not lend themselves to a moment's experience. An example might be the loss of our youth, surely inevitable, but who can give it a precise time and setting? Personal losses that which may have meaning only in the context of one individual's life and story are beyond the scope of a traditional imperative. And yet all of our losses require attention, not only those specifically referenced in the pages of rabbinic wisdom. It has become increasingly clear to me over the years of attending to the sick and infirm that caregiving needs to take its cue more from the model of *nichum aveilim*, comforting the mourner, than from *bikur cholim*, visiting the sick. Frequently, an essential spiritual issue the person we meet at the bedside is confronting is one of loss. We who provide care must see ourselves as visitors to the bereaved. Our conduct, manner, and method would be most effective if we model ourselves in the image of one making a *shiva* visit.

That said, it needs to be clear that to the extent we are fearful of confronting our own losses we will fail to visit effectively the sick and help them confront theirs. If the caregiver, be he/she chaplain or other, has avoided the painful in his/her own life, like Ruth in our earlier example, then he/she will not be able to sit with another and help him/her grieve. Typically, the chaplain will excuse an unwillingness to sit with the patient's lament with the words "Why should I make him/her feel worse?" Truth be told, it is not the patient's needs the chaplain is considering. If the good of the other was motivating the chaplain, it would be clear from the tradition of the *shiva* visit that the only way through a loss is to grieve it. We need to experience our separations in order to find comfort and re-attach. What motivates the chaplain to avoid the loss is rather his/her own fear to confront the losses in his/her life. It is because he/she has struggled to find the courage to do the work of separation with its attendant grief that he/she finds reason to avoid joining the other in his/her work of grief. Not only does the caregiver not help the patient in a time of great need. He/she by skirting the loss and its consequences delivers a message, not unlike Ruth's mother in our earlier story, that acknowledging loss will cause irreparable suffering, rather than impart the truth, that experiencing it in its fullness is the way to healing and rebirth.

I do not mean to imply that to be a good caregiver one needs to have entirely processed one's losses. The work of separation with its attendant grief and attachment with its attendant hope are lifelong. We are always in some form or other coming to new expressions of grief even as we mature and understand earlier losses in new ways. We may have had a parent die when we were twenty-five and mourn as we knew how at that time. Still when we reach fifty and are in search of counsel we may experience the loss of that same parent again, and in a new way, and around a new sense of how we might have so much needed them now. What the caregiver must possess is the courage to face his/her own losses, to be willing to sit with them, cry the tears, experience the hurt. The caregiver must believe in the value of grief-work him/herself if he/she is to effectively companion another in that sacred work.

It is important here to make clear what exactly the work of separation is about. How do we come to process our losses? What does it mean to help another in that effort? Let us refer to our own tradition to show us the method. In the aftermath of a death, the immediate family are mandated to spend a week in mourning referred to as *shiva*. During that week, the mourners live with their loss. All of life's activities, from the morning shave (forbidden) to the change of clothes (forbidden), are experienced in the context of the loss. The mourner stays at home during the week and waits on his/her grief, waits for the tears, waits for the stories, waits for the feelings to come. Community members come and visit during the week. They are present to listen, and invite the mourners to share with another the tears, the stories, the feelings that arise. At times, the visitor may share a story of his/her own concerning the loved one who died with the goal of helping the mourner appreciate even more fully the significance of his/her loss. What is made clear from tradition is that to grieve is to become fully conscious of what one had so that one can experience its absence. The more one is aware of the gift that was present to them in the life of the parent/sibling/spouse/child taken from them, the more he/she will experience loss and its attendant feelings. Rather than run from them, we must experience them in their fullness for healing to happen and new attachments made possible.

When visiting the sick and infirmed, who like the mourning are experiencing loss – loss of dreams, loss of expectations, loss of role, loss of status, to name but a few of the kinds of losses illness brings on – the caregiver needs to help by inviting expression of the loss. The sick person needs to be able to speak in detail of what he/she once had and now does not. He/she needs to be able to tell the stories of what was true in the past and is now gone. When we visit a woman who because of her condition is soon to be moved out of her home and into a geriatric facility, we need to anticipate the visit in the framework of a *shiva* visit. In hearing the woman's sadness, we need to help her talk about the home she is losing. We might ask, "What was your favorite room?" "What kind of furniture did you have?" "What are your favorite memories of good times had in your home?" We need to realize that talking about loss is not talking about the absence. Rather, it is remembering what it is that one is now separated from in all its detail and meaning. To grieve is to tell stories, the stories of that which was, so as to become most conscious of the impact of its absence.

Not all losses are alike. Indeed experts in the field of grief and loss have come to recognize different categories of loss. Kenneth R. Mitchell and Herbert Anderson in their book *All Our Losses, All Our Griefs: Resources for Pastoral Care* distinguish several kinds of loss. Briefly, some of those include:

(1) *Material loss*, which refers to the loss of something material, say the loss of money in a stock devaluation;

(2) *Relationship loss*, which we most commonly associate with the death of a person important to us in relationship;

(3) *Role loss*, which refers to the loss of one's position in the context of family or perhaps society, say when the father is now dependent on his children for care;

(4) *Function loss*, when one's ability to do certain things is compromised, say when one can no longer get around independently;

(5) *Intrapsychic loss*, which refers to the loss of one's sense of who one is, the disappointment in one's failure to be the person one expected oneself to be.[8]

8. Kenneth R. Mitchell and Herbert Anderson, *All Our Losses, All Our Griefs: Resources for Pastoral Care* (Philadelphia, Westminster Press, 1983) p 36ff

What is important to recognize in identifying kinds of losses is that to help another give expression to his/her loss one must first understand what it is exactly he/she is grieving. I can remember Ari, a rabbi in his mid-thirties, a student in my CPE program, who came into the group one morning devastated. When asked about his state of mind, he shared that his car had been stolen over the weekend. He was overwhelmed with grief. At first his peers and I struggled to comprehend the loss. "Yes," he said, he had insurance. "No," it was an older car, not really of great value. So what was bothering Ari so much? Only with time did we come to realize that Ari's loss of the car was not a "material loss" but a "relationship loss." The car, he explained, was given to him by his father as a graduation gift from seminary five years earlier. It represented his father's acceptance of his career choice and affirmation of his gifts after years of struggle. Only on understanding what the loss of his car meant to him could we offer Ari the community of comforters to successfully help him grieve and separate.

Each person's loss is unique to them in the context of his/her life and consistent with the makeup of his/her personality. Often professionals in the field speak of anticipatory grief to characterize a person's feelings around their own demise or the soon-to-be death of a loved one. When visiting a person who is coming to grips with his/her approaching death, whether that death will come in a day, a week, a month, or sometimes not for many years, we need to accept the grief and sadness attendant to the loss experience. We also need to recognize that at times other feelings are present, including anger, guilt, and fear. Loss is not something that can be measured in objective terms. We cannot, for example, say to the forty-five-year-old man who has learned he has kidney disease that he need not grieve because in light of recent medical advances he will likely be able to live a long time with the disease. While that may be true, the man with the disease needs to experience his loss, whatever it may be, perhaps an intrapsychic loss, as he has to reimage himself as a wounded person, or a loss of dreams, perhaps that he would play basketball at eighty-five with his grandchildren. For this man something has died in his new medical condition. In order for this man to live the remainder of his life successfully, he needs to first grieve that which is gone and separate from it. This will allow him to attach to a new reality and begin life with an appreciation for the gifts and opportunities now available to him. In order for this man to live fully in the present circumstances and be true to himself and his life story he will need to let go of what is no more and keep it alive in memory. He will need companions who will sit with him and support him as he does that meaningful and difficult work. These companions need to know that his sadness is not depression nor is it bad. On the contrary, the sadness and other feelings that may arise including anger, impatience, selfishness, fear, to name a few, are part of the process of grieving that will in the end bring the one they care for through to the other side where new relationships are born. Trusting the one we care for and trust of the process are the most important ingredients for good caregiving in the aftermath of loss.

Jewish tradition intimates in a very striking way the truth of the process of grief and recovery we have been discussing. In the Hebrew language the word for comfort is *nachama*. To comfort is *l'nachem*. The root three letters of the verb are *nun*, *chet* and *mem*. Those letters and indeed the verb itself also have another meaning. In Hebrew, "*l'nachem*" is to experience change. For example, when the Torah describes God's decision to destroy humanity at the time of the Deluge, God said "because *nichamti* that I have made them..."[9], meaning God had regret, or better, had a change of attitude (direction) about creation. A similar use of the three-letter verb occurs at the time of the worship of the Golden Calf, where God initially was determined to destroy the Israelites. After Moses' petition the verse reads, "*Vayenachem Hashem al haraah asher dibber lasot l'amo.*"[10] God changed God's attitude (direction) about the evil He had intended to do to God's people. The word for change is *vayenachem*, with the same three root letters, *nun*, *chet* and *mem*. We might well wonder about the relationship between the three-letter root *nun*, *chet*, *mem* meaning both comfort

9. Genesis 6:7
10. Exodus 32:14

and change in a language in which similarities of construct imply similarities of concept.

In light of our earlier discussion, the message implied in the He-brew usage can be understood. For indeed to experience comfort is to go through an experience of change of direction. *Nachama* comes about not by forgetting one's loss or minimizing it. Rather for comfort to happen one has to enter into it deeply, feel its full impact, live its truth. When one has lived the story of loss and done the work of grieving something remarkable happens. The very same energy that engendered the emotional response to sepa-ration becomes transformed to provide the stimulus to healing and new attachment. That which fuels the one fuels the other. The movement from grief to comfort is a redirection of the same life energy flowing through the human psyche. To be comforted is not to gain something new or to lose something old, but rather to expe-rience redirection of the current from that focused on the absence to that focused on the opportunity. Failure to find comfort needs to be understood as an absence of that life energy. If it is withheld in grief, it will not be available to be transformed into the elixir of comfort. Indeed, *nun-chet-mem* means both comfort and change of direction, because the latter is the way to the former.

No matter how one spells comfort, in the face of loss comfort requires another. The friend, the spouse, the rabbi, the profession-al caregiver are necessary to provide the invitation to the griev-ing to enter their loss in story and feeling. Moreover the other in entering the world of the grieving provides the confidence to the mourner that he/she will come out of the process intact, and that he/she need not worry about losing him/herself in the sadness that he/she will not come out the other side. In the knowing nod of the caregiver who watches and listens as the grieving one expresses him/herself, the caregiver gives assurance that letting go with its attendant hurt is the path that is both necessary and vital to life restored. Real loving, that which is a true expression of following in the ways of the Divine, the source for our responsibility to do *hesed*, does not express itself in protecting the suffering from facing their losses. Rather, real loving is manifest in our capacity to sit with the hurting other in his/her loss knowing that thereby he/she will in the end come to the new attachments life will offer with all their promise and meaning.

Chapter 10
Between Hope and Despair

> When the sun set on the very day Adam was created,
> he said, "Perhaps it is because of my wrongdoing that the
> world is going dark, and it will be returned once again to
> emptiness and confusion. Perhaps this is the death that
> Heaven condemned me to suffer."
>
> He fasted and cried through the night and Eve cried
> opposite him. When the dawn came, Adam said, "This
> is the way of the world." He rose and offered an ox for a
> sacrifice.[1]

Despair can be described as one's experience of his/her world going dark. It is an unbearable feeling and one that cannot be lived in for long. Typically, when we have an experience of despair, say when we fail in an effort to secure a new job that was important to us or when we disappoint our parents and recognize we have failed to meet their life's expectations of us, we sigh deeply; we feel an overwhelming depletion of energy; we may cry; we may lash out wildly. When feeling despair we often feel small, powerless, overwhelmed. In response to the feeling of despair, we often tend to run. We run at times to safer harbors, to focus on other parts of our lives that are not black. We may run to escape in sleep or other mind-numbing behaviors. We may run by immersing ourselves in self-destructive indulgences, such as alcohol abuse and binge eating. The term that most

---

1. Avoda Zarah 8a

connotes the feeling of despair is surrender. In despair we surrender to our circumstances. We give up, resigned to the fate we feel we cannot escape.

It is important here that we distinguish between despair and depression. Despair is a spiritual term. It reflects a malaise of the soul. It is a direct response to one's circumstances and the meaning one has attached to them. Its characteristic is a pervasive sense of emptiness. Depression is not a spiritual struggle but a psychological disease. To speak of someone as depressed is to make an assessment of his/her psychological state. Often depression has been defined as decontextualized grief, that is, a grief not a response to a specific loss but rather taken on as an internalized way of being in the world. Depression may have its roots in an event. It may have been triggered by a specific loss or tragedy. But to the extent depression is diagnosed the feelings, which may have first been associated with loss, have become planted in the psyche.

Mental health professionals diagnose and treat depression. As caregivers we respond to despair. Too often, caregivers, be they rabbis, chaplains, friends, or family, are quick to label someone's manner as depression, their condition as depressed. That frees them of responsibility and makes the case for medical intervention. Still more often mental health professionals are quick to label the spiritual issues of grief and despair as depression. They then medicate the disease rather than respond to the person and his/her struggle.

Unlike depression, despair is not a disease. It is an existential struggle with life and its challenges. It is a noble struggle, heroic at times. In response to despair, one does not so much need medication as one needs to discover meaning and hope. In one's despair one feels not emotionally dead or disconnected from self as in the experience of depression. On the contrary, in despair one feels alive, in touch with one's core yearnings even as those yearnings have been thwarted. As in the story of Adam's first night with which we opened the chapter, in one's despair one often cries, fasts, expresses a fullness of emotion. In fact, the tendency to flee from despair, as we discussed above, is a flight from the intensity of the feeling, a feeling we can't help but acknowledge and yet at the same time struggle to accept.

To help us reflect on the experience of despair and in turn hope, let me share from the writing of Milton Graub, a professor of pediatrics at Hahneman Medical College in Philadelphia, as he wrote about his experience with his own daughter Kathy, when he learned she had cystic fibrosis.

"How can anyone relate how he really feels after the death of an eighteen-year-old daughter, a child so beautiful in soul, delicate in mind, and so loving to all? The task is almost unbearable.

"I will never forget the night I spoke to Evelyn, my wife, who was with our ill daughter, Kathy, then age two. Evelyn informed me not only that the results of Kathy's duodenal drainage tests were positive but also that Kathy had cystic fibrosis. (Almost two years earlier the same diagnosis had been established for our infant son.) It was 1951. I was a young and optimistic pediatric resident just beginning to learn something about this 'rare and fatal disease.' My words to my wife were simple and straightforward: we must be strong and have faith; we would do all we could for our children and beyond this we could do nothing more. This attempt to support Evelyn, and the support she gave me, became a way of life for both of us; without it I am not sure that we could have survived the following sixteen years.

"My first real feelings of depression and despair occurred that night. I was alone and cried most of the night. The future seemed almost hopeless; to have had two children both with this dread disease was incomprehensible to me. Every other problem I had ever faced could be rationalized and, with persistence and work, some reasonable answer could be found. But I could see no positive outcome from my current plight, no matter where or how my thoughts turned.

"My despair finally took the form of compromise: compromise in the knowledge that I had a wonderful wife and that we could still be a small, happy family. In my youth and innocence, I had not yet experienced how beautiful children, well *or sick*, can be. And I had not yet come to know that life is just a series of memories after all.

"Kathy did fairly well until the age of eight, when she developed her first serious pulmonary infection. I had been fairly relaxed until then, enjoying her every experience with her. It was at this time that I was brought harshly back to reality. It had been my policy to leave all health decisions to Kathy's pediatrician, not even asking him the results of her laboratory studies. However, when she was hospitalized with this infection, I saw her radiographs and for the first time realized that she was showing typical progressive changes of the disease. Prior to this, she had been attending school daily, enjoying vacations with us, and was well-nourished. I had shut out the true progressive nature of the disease, and when confronted by the objective evidence of the radiograph films I was shattered, and re-experienced the despair, depression, and hopelessness that I had felt when she was an infant and the initial diagnosis had been made.

"Time and her presence again were my immediate salvation. The next ten years were years of great love, delight, and growth, both for Evelyn and for me. Kathy taught us so many things: how to be appreciative of each day; how, in spite of deficiencies, to adapt and make the best of a situation. She loved baseball, went out for her school softball team each year (though she didn't make it, since she couldn't even run to first base). But in trying she taught us how to be positive and look at life in a more humorous vein; and, above all, to be brave in the face of a life of medications, treatments, and the all-pervasive knowledge of cystic fibrosis.

"The above qualities, together with a wonderful ability to show affection, made her a very special person to us; and so, when Kathy became critically ill, I initially could not accept the idea she might die. She had been sick so many times before and had always responded to treatment. It was not until the day that her dedicated physician indicated to me that she was in cardiac failure and was not responding that I realized the truth. Even though I knew how little functioning lung tissue remained, and could see her peripheral edema, only upon being told by someone else did I fully realize that our Kathy was dying. Denial had been the only defense, and now it failed.

"I could not control myself. I stayed with her all that day and wept continuously. I simply could not understand how we could bear not to have her with us. Her problems, her therapy, and her limitations had become an integral part of our daily existence. They had become normal focus and no burden on the family. How could this large part of our existence suddenly disappear and life remain whole?

"Kathy spoke infrequently that day but continued to open her eyes to see if we were there. She seldom smiled and once, seeing my tears, asked why I was crying. I believe she had always maintained such a positive outlook that she actually didn't realize that she could be dying.

I couldn't find a comfortable place that day or night. I paced and wept, saying little. My mind was numb but groped for some basis upon which I might continue living without her. I believe my feelings added up to a total of 'nothingness.'

"Kathy died the next morning. Although I did not feel that she had been relieved of her suffering and was, therefore, better off, I was consoled by the thought that she had lived a full, happy, and intellectually active life. It was also consoling to know that as parents, we had loved her, that this love had been returned, and that we had done all that was humanly possible for her.

"She knew how deeply involved our family was with the cystic fibrosis cause and I think she always believed that because of efforts such as ours, the "control" would come in time to help *her*. This thought supported her to the end

"We lived the 'Impossible Dream.'"[2]

The father's story has its similarities to the story of Adam with which we began the chapter. On learning of Kathy's diagnosis, Milton's despair is manifest in an outpouring of emotion. He wept; he vented; he gave painful voice to his thwarted dreams both for

---

2. Milton Graub, *The Thoughts of a Bereaved Father* in *Anticipatory Grief*, Bernard Schoenberg, Arthur C. Carr, Austin H. Kutscher, David Peretz, Ivan Goldberg (editors), (New York and London, Columbia University Press, 1974) pp 158-161

himself and his family. It is also a story of hope. At each stage of Kathy's life, Milton found hope in the aftermath of despair, albeit a hope narrowed by the realities of the dreams denied. In fact, real hope is forever the gift discovered only through the dark night of despair. When Adam in our opening Midrash saw the light of dawn he said, "This is the way of the world." Yet how did he know that to be true after only one night? Moreover, he only saw the dawn. He did not yet see the sunrise. How did he know the light in its fullness would return? Truth is, Adam did not know that this was the way of the world with any degree of certainty. And yet after his journey through the despair he saw the dawn as his hope, and he embraced its possibilities as a source for engaging life once again.

As providers of care, we often enter the world of those experiencing despair. We meet the family in their hours of pervasive darkness, when they feel what they most hoped for has been denied. In response typically we try to offer hope. We share some information we hope the others will embrace as a beacon of light to dispel their darkness. Most often hope brought in from outside has little impact on the suffering. They hear the words. They might even want to believe them, but the hope does not last. We leave the rooms and an hour later the heaviness is back in full measure. In truth, the hope we offered was but a diversion from the struggle. Real hope, hope that offers promise for meaning in the face of surrender, emerges only through the struggle and only in the hearts of those living and searching for the light.

Let's look as the case of Milton and imagine ourselves as caregivers to him, whether as chaplains, rabbis, or friends. Upon learning that Kathy, his daughter, had cystic fibrosis, we would be enormously sad for him and his family. We would have our own battle not to be overwhelmed with despair. We would struggle to imagine how Milton might find hope in the face of such tragic circumstances. On our entering the scene with Milton what might we say? We might try to tell him to have faith, that God will take care of Kathy and the family and who knows, cure is always possible. We might say something like "Science/medicine doesn't always have it right."

We might tell him, "Don't give up. There's alwe
in our own hearts we would know we were (
trying to overcome our own despair by proviu.
not believe. Since we don't have to live with Kathy da,
out, these empty expressions of hope might work for us. It an.
us to go home and eat dinner with out family. But for Milton, who
lives with Kathy, words of "wishes" are not the same as "hope." He
needs a dose of hope, one he can live with day to day in the midst
of the devastating prognosis and the developing story.

What Milton would need from us is to enter his world and sit
with him in the despair. Listen to his cry. Hear the heroic journey
he is on to ultimately find something to hold on to when all feels
lost. In truth, isn't that what happened to Milton? At each stage of
Kathy's life and story Milton found hope, different hope to be sure,
different in light of the changing circumstances. But in the end it
was those real hopes adjusted through each defeat that helped him
persevere and even grow as a person through a horrible tragedy. If
anyone had told Milton when he first heard Kathy's diagnosis to
find hope in compromise, as he later described the process, to accept the beauty of what he had rather than focus on what he did
not, that person would not only have been unhelpful, they likely
would have elicited anger. Even the hope ultimately realized feels
punishing when offered by someone outside the experience and at
a premature time. The caregiver's work is to sit in the darkness
with the despairing one, to allow them their dark night of the soul,
and to trust that if we stay the course, he/she will find what he/she
needs to reclaim life in the midst of his/her disappointment.

In order to care for someone else in the midst of his/her despair,
we need to have our own hope for the suffering one we are minis-
tering to. We need to have a vision of what might be possible for
him/her. Unless we have hope ourselves, we will be unable to sit
with the suffering in their time of surrender. We will either avoid
them or offer platitudes so as not to confront the hopelessness ourselves. Having a vision of what the other side of despair might look
like for a parent who has to confront the inevitable in the death
of a child is vital to giving us the ability to walk with that parent

and trust he/she can find his/her way through. The hope we have for him/her may not be the hope he/she ultimately embraces, but as long as we have a hope we can tolerate the despair of the other and support him/her in the struggle. As caregivers we must sit ourselves in the darkness of the other's story to find some true and meaningful hope for him/her. Not that we share that hope with the other. No, the other must discover hope for him/herself. But so that we can trust the process believing hope is indeed possible, for alas we have seen an expression of it. We can now comfortably hope the other will find their hope, for there is indeed hope to be found.

Let's explore the world of hope in the face of tragedy. What does meaningful hope look like? What can we as caregivers hope that the suffering will find in the midst of even the most devastating of circumstances to sustain them? I can remember the story of Craig, a Jewish man in his early thirties who was dying from AIDS. His last stay in the hospital where I was chaplain was long and torturous. He suffered physical pain and had a great sense of emotional/spiritual diminishment. Craig wanted to die. He called the hospice team to plan for the cessation of nutrition and hydration. If he could not eat by mouth he wanted no tube feedings any longer. I was present as he addressed the team. It was a sad and tragic time. Yet Craig was adamant that the hospice team not take over his care until Thursday, and this was Monday. It was puzzling why he insisted on waiting four days. Later Craig explained. He said the massage therapists came around the hospital on Wednesday. His one pleasure was the back massage he received from the therapists. It brought him a sense of feeling cared for. Even in his plans for death he insisted on this last pleasure. It was this hope, limited though it was, that made life desirable for Craig's last days even amid a certain and debilitating death.

For many, hope is not some transcendent yearning or a great victory over their circumstances. Rather hope may be just an improvement over the situation of the present. Menachem Begin was imprisoned by the Communists in Russia in the 1930s. In his autobiography, *Revolt*, he described the horrific conditions of his incarceration. He wrote that his dreams in the jail cell were not that he be able to lay in a sumptuously decorated room on a thick down-filled mattress. All his hope was that he have some straw to lay on rather than be resigned to the bare hard floor.[3] Frequently in listening to the voices of the sick and suffering, we hear a similar refrain. They hope not for the great deliverance that seems too distant and beyond even their imagination. They hope for no pain today, or just the chance to go home one more time, or to see the birth of their grandchild. Sometimes, like Craig, they simply hope for a simple pleasure.

These hopes need to be nourished by the chaplain or other caregiver. They may seem trite, but they help the sick and suffering get through one day at a time. In the language of Hassidic mysticism, we might call this *katnut d'mochin*, the limited consciousness, that is, the person's way of experiencing the world out of his/her more confined sense of self. In *katnut d'mochin*, a person is acutely aware of his/her finitude and his/her existence as limited to the time and space of the present. To speak to another of the transcendent when he/she is in the midst of *katnut d'mochin* is unproductive. Rather the conversation needs to honor the mindset of the one in travail, and hope needs to be expressed in the context of his/her state of consciousness.

And yet at a deep level we who care for and love another hope that he/she will find a more sustaining hope, one that will endure beyond the limitations of any given day or circumstance. We want to believe that in the midst of even the most devastating tragedy a hope can be born that will not only serve as a life raft in a stormy sea but will truly bring a measure of light into the darkness. We know that no hope we can imagine will ever turn the story from a tragedy to a comedy and yet we want to find a hope that at least will give the tragedy meaning and give the struggle of the suffering a sense of purpose. While we do not have the end of Milton's story before us in his write-up, indeed this was part of his expanding hope. After Kathy's death, Milton went on to become involved still more closely in the American Association for Cystic Fibrosis,

---

3. Menachem Begin, *Revolt* (New York, E.P. Dutton, 1978)

ultimately becoming its president. While he could not save Kathy, he gave her story meaning by using it to impel him to care and seek cure for others. He wrote and lectured. He raised consciousness of both the disease and the need for a response. This hope born in Milton would be referred to in the Hassidic mystical literature as *gadlut d'mochin*, or the expanded sense of consciousness. It is the hope born out of Milton's sense of himself as in some ways tran-scendent, belonging to a larger community of humankind, maybe even being in-part-connected to the eternal. *Gadlut d'mochin*, when one is in touch with the self in an expanded sense, leads to a hope that provides meaning and gives life purpose. In one's state of *gadlut d'mochin*, one can find an ultimate hope, a hope that will neither pass with time nor be limited to a set of circumstances. It is the hope of the human when he/she is most in touch with the essence of who he/she is.

The difference between *gadlut d'mochin* and *katnut d'mochin* is the difference between Milton and Craig and their respective hopes. Each faced a situation he could not defeat. Each expe-rienced despair. In Milton's case the despair led to a hope that was both transcendent and expansive. Most importantly in Craig's case his suffering caused him to remain constricted, even with his hope. The hope did not move him beyond his broken sense of self. In Milton's case through the hope he grew larger than the awful-ness of his predicament. On the wings of his hope he outgrew the shadow that enveloped him. Such is the power of hope in its most profound expression. Hope in its most meaningful form does not merely help us survive our circumstance. Hope in that form sus-tains us. That hope becomes our life.

In a profound way it is the hope of *gadlut d'mochin* that we as caregivers help engender in the other by patiently living with him/her in his/her despair. Through steadfastly supporting the parent whose child died and who feels lost and empty through the months of "emptiness," we help him/her find a hope that could not emerge in a day or a week. We help him/her find a hope transcendent, one that may well reshape his/her life. Those whose tragedies have led them to new life missions inevitably were sustained in their despair so that they could come to the kind of hope that could only emerge once ripened through tears and time. So many of the great contributions to society have been generated by individuals who sustained tragedy and who later responded with passion to forge new blessings, their hope expressed in making creative change. Whatever the change that hope produces in the person or in the world he/she inhabits, we need to know it could not occur without a winter of despair.

For the faithful, one may hope that through their suffering and despair they may find hope through a deeper bond with God. In the liturgy we recite the verse, "In thy deliverance I hope O Lord"[4], a verse of three Hebrew words, over and over three times, flipping each time the sequence of the words into three different permutations. We express those three versions of the call to hope on several occasions, once at the very end of the morning service, after we have recited the "six remembrances" and the thirteen principles of faith of Maimonides. At that time we not only say the three verses of hope in the original Hebrew form. We also recite it in Aramaic, and again here in all three permutations. The same three verses in the Hebrew form are recited in the prayer at bedtime, and for some in the traveler's prayer. The call to hope in God for the religious is the response to the potential despair that the day's challenges may bring, or that may come in the dark night of sleep and dreaming, or that may occur on the road. Knowing that we can hope for God's deliverance even when our own circumstances may shout defeat gives us courage and calls on us to confront the world with less fear of despair. Hope for God's deliverance is an expression of *gadlut d'mochin* that we can aspire to only through the inspiration of the morning prayers when we have had the experience of intimacy with the Divine. Even then we repeat the call to hope over and over almost as a mantra to rouse ourselves to the spiritual within us so we might embrace its transcendent call.

Those for whom faith has less meaning may find a hope transcendent but more personal in nature. A wonderful example can be seen in Harper Lee's classic *To Kill a Mockingbird*. In one of

4. Genesis 49:18

the book's more poignant vignettes, Atticus's twelve-year-old son, Jem, was compelled to visit with Mrs. Dubose, a cantankerous old woman whose prize bushes he had clipped in reaction to her abusive and insulting manner. Mrs. Dubose was cancer-ridden and arthritic. Jem had to read to her each day at her bedside for a month. Some time after the penance was completed, Atticus was summoned to Mrs. Dubose's home. When he returned late that night, he and Jem had this conversation.

"She's dead, son," said Atticus. "She died a few minutes ago."

"Oh," said Jem. "Well."

"Well is right," said Atticus. She's not suffering any more. She was sick for a long time. Son, didn't you know what those fits were?"

Jem shook his head.

"Mrs. Dubose was a morphine addict," said Atticus. "She took it as a pain killer for years. The doctor put her on it. She'd have spent the rest life on it and died without so much agony, but she was too contrary –"

"Sir?" said Jem.

"She said she was going to leave this world beholden to nothing and nobody. Jem, when you're sick as she was, it's all right to take anything to make it easier, but it wasn't all right for her. She said she meant to break herself of it before she died and that's what she did."

"…Did she die free?" asked Jem.

"As the mountains air," said Atticus. "She was conscious to the last almost. Conscious," he smiled, "and cantankerous. …I wanted you to see something about her. I wanted you to see what real courage is, instead of getting the idea that courage is a man with a gun in his hand. It's when you know you're licked before you begin but you begin anyway and you see it through no matter what. You rarely win, but sometimes you do. Mrs. Dubose won, all ninety-eight pounds of her. According to her views she died beholden to nothing and nobody. She was the bravest person I ever knew."[5]

For many who face the feelings of despair over and over again in being defeated by a chronic and pernicious illness, the hope may well be that through it all they will remain their authentic selves. No, still more, they will, through the process, become more their authentic selves. The ultimate hope for many can be expressed as, "No matter what, I will be me." Knowing like Mrs. Dubose that they can be true to themselves no matter how damaging the disease or severe life's persecution is the one great triumph that offers meaning to existence and unconditional hope.

In closing this chapter let us read the words of the Psalmist who in one of the most familiar of Psalms, the *Shir Hamalot*, the Song of Ascents, recited before the blessings after the meal on Sabbaths and holidays poignantly expresses the journey from despair to hope as a process with each part vital to the other.

In writing of the returnees of the exiles the Psalmist compares them to a farmer. "Those who sow in tears will reap with joyful song. [Though] he walks along weeping carrying a bag of seed, he will return with joyous song carrying his sheaves."[6] It is the tears, the weeping of the one in despair broken and compromised, that holds in its expression the promise of redemption and hope. The sacred work of caregiving in the face of despair is to support these tears, to sustain the other in his/her weeping so indeed the joy to them may come.

In the Hebrew language the word for hope, *kaveh*, also means to wait. Indeed as we have discussed to find real hope is to have the courage to wait, to live in the emptiness, trusting that a hope authentic and transcendent will yet come to usher in the dawn. "Wait in the Lord; be of good courage and He shall strengthen thine heart; wait, I say, in the Lord."[7]

---

5. Harper Lee, *To Kill a Mockingbird* (New York, Popular Library, 1962) pp 115-116

6. Psalms 126: 5-6

7. Psalms 27:4

Chapter 11
Knowing Thyself

I was serving a mostly older congregation in Wilkes Barre, Pennsylvania. My pastoral responsibilities and my own investment in caregiving led me to several units of Clinical Pastoral Education, all at regional medical centers. I felt I found my call in the rabbinate and it was to respond to the marginalized and infirm, not through social action but through offering healing relationship. Perhaps then it was no big surprise to my synagogue president, a man of similar age and a lawyer by profession, when I visited him in his office one morning with my request.

"Murray," I said, "I want to spend three days each week working at a large medical center in New York City. In addition to being your rabbi, I want to be a chaplain. And I am asking you to let me follow my dream of caring for the hurting and the sick."

Murray looked into my eyes and responded, "Rabbi, I know you feel a need to care for the sick. We will have to discuss your proposal with the synagogue leadership and see what we can do."

In the end, I never did pursue that arrangement with the synagogue. Instead, I left the congregation and moved to New York City to begin my journey to become a certified supervisor of Clinical Pastoral Education. But what remained for me from that encounter was Murray's comment, "I know you feel a need..." Though he never knew it, I was in fact startled and upset by his observation. What did he mean, "I know you feel a need..."? My sense of my request was that it evidenced my compassion, my altruism, my deep identification with the hurting. It was not for me about "my" need but about the needs of those less fortunate than I. What Murray had done was take that of which I was most proud and frame it simply as an expression of my psychic makeup. It was as if he was saying, "Some may need to make money; you need to visit patients."

Over time I came to realize exactly how right Murray was. My investment in providing care was not indeed some expression of a higher self, a commitment to others that reflected a more noble personality. My commitment to caring emerged out of my need to be needed, a dimension of my personality whose source I have both come to understand and appreciate. I cannot rightfully view myself as some noble character, committed to the welfare of others, and see myself as above those whose lives are involved in more clearly defined self-serving pursuits, such as making money. I, too, am essentially involved in a self-serving pursuit, only my self-pursuit manifests itself in providing care. That's where I get my needs met.

I have begun this final chapter not with a story from tradition as in our other chapters but with a self-story. That is because this chapter is about ourselves as caregivers. And to be a good caregiver we must know ourselves. Caregiving is not a work like cabinet-making or systems programming. In most professions, it does not matter what one's intentions are in doing the work. It is the objective realized that is of import. The man filling my gas tank can be imagining at the time he is stuffing his turkey, it matters not at all. Even caregiving when it involves the performance of a physical gesture does not really require self-awareness. The poor man does not care much if in giving him the hundred dollars I am looking for gratitude or needing to feel superior. He has the money for his rent in any case. The nurse at the time he/she is giving the injection may feel love toward the patient or resentment over her job. It will matter little if the patient receives the fluids vital for his/her recovery.

Caregiving in the context we have discussed through the book, however, is at its core about relationship. And in relationship intentions do matter. Whereas for other life endeavors and even in other forms of caregiving the what of the activity is the central concern, in the form of caregiving through relationship we have been discussing, the why matters every bit as much as the what. And unless one knows why one is doing what one is doing, he/she is at risk of not only compromising the helping act but in fact causing the other harm.

The examples of helpers being unaware of their motivations and causing harm are legion. In its simple forms, we need only think of the parent who protects the child by removing life's challenges as in the case of Ruth in Chapter Nine. You may recall her mother hid from her the death of her father. That led to Ruth's lifelong avoidance of intimacy. To be sure Ruth's mother thought she was caring for Ruth. In fact she was responding to her own inability to see her child grieve. Boundary violations are a frequent problem for helpers who get their own needs met while claiming an idealistic zeal, in fact too often not helping but compromising the vulnerable other. Maxine Glaz in an article titled "Reconstructing the Pastoral Care of Women" tells of the compassionate clergyperson whose helping initiatives with several women who had come to an awareness of early childhood sexual molestation led to successive suicides. In each case, he invited the women to share their story. He was an attentive listener, available, comforting. He thought he was helping. Yet he allowed each to visit him at off-hours and more frequently than the norm. Each felt in the end not helped but compromised, in a relationship without boundaries, again vulnerable to an authority. The clergyman thought he was responding to the needs of the hurting women. Only later did he come to realize that it was his need to care that governed his motivation and with tragic consequences.[1] While the above case may seem the extreme, on clinical review the amount of damage done in the guise of helping is enormous and most often unrecognized. Almost all of it can be attributed to the unconscious needs of the helper being imposed upon the unsuspecting and needy helpee.

Let me be still more specific. While I am now aware of my

---

1. Maxine Glaz, "Reconstructing the Pastoral Care of Women" in *Second Opinion*, October 1991

own need to be needed as the source of my desire to help, I could not say I was conscious of that for many years. My own need to be heroic with those who were struggling with life's circumstances at times led me to coddle people who would have been better off challenged. I know my "niceness" kept them stuck in a dependent situation. Yes, I massaged their hurts, but they would have been better off stimulated to make the changes necessary to move out of the victim mode. Yet I liked feeling like I was caring and needed. I felt good about myself for what I offered even as nothing changed for them. It would have been better if I had recognized my need to be appreciated and then let it go, in order to do what would truly have been best for the hurting other, even if they would not have known it in the moment.

In truth my story, the tragic story of the compassionate clergyman and all other similar stories we could tell, reveal a simple reality. No one, and I mean no one, ever does anything for another simply for the benefit of the other. There is no true altruism. Caregiving at its best is done because we find pleasure in seeing another cared for. We give charity, we do favors, we raise children all because it makes us happy to do it. In the purest sense, that happiness is derived from our love for the other. In more compromised motivation, we help others for the realization of more personal needs, in my case the need to be needed, in other cases to win respect and admiration, in still others in order to fix unfinished business in our families of origin. Let me share some of the thinking theorists in the field have uncovered as to that which motivates clergy to choose caregiving as the focus of their vocation.

Allen Wheelis many years ago theorized that those who choose a profession that calls for involvement with the inner life of others and the provision of care are strongly influenced by a desire to alleviate inner conflicts within themselves. He argued that the choice of a career in caregiving is typically rooted in the unconscious desire of the caregiver to work out issues arising in their family of origin.[2] What issues are they? Some suggest that caregivers

---

2. Allen Wheelis, *The Quest for Identity* (New York, W.W. Norton, 1958) pp 206ff

are influenced by the need to compensate for the unfinished business of their family system. Take, for example, the father who had hoped to become a rabbi but because of a hardship, say the family's financial plight, was unable to realize that call and instead ran the family business. His child may unconsciously take on the father's sense of incompleteness and attempt to redress the unfairness of the family script by becoming the "rabbi" for his father. It is not out of his own personal desire that the child, now adult, chooses, in this example, the profession of the rabbinate. In fact, he may really want to be a college history professor. But without really knowing it, he adopts the family's agenda and assumes the career choice not chosen in the earlier generation. He believes the choice to be a rabbi is his truest desire and often only later, frequently at mid-life, and often through a crisis, comes to realize that the choice was not in truth consistent with his deepest self.[3]

Others have suggested different family of origin scripts. In some scenarios, caregivers are typically parentified as children. They for one reason or another have been oriented into the role of caregiving from their youth. Sometimes it is an overt role of caregiver they take on, as in cases where they are the oldest children and one or both of the parents are not able to function properly due to physical or emotional impairment. In those cases, they may be providing care for younger siblings or even the parents themselves from their youth. Sometimes the parentification of the child is more covert. The caregivers as children respond unconsciously to the limited capacities of their parents to meet their needs and those of their siblings. They become intent on being "good" children, never requiring attention, always with the goal of making mom and dad proud. They are busy working in their homes to bring the kind of stability and support that will allow a more compromised parent to function.[4] In a variation on that script, some have understood the profile of the caregiver as developing in him/

3. Ivan Boszormenyi-Nagy and Geraldine M. Spark, *Invisible Loyalties: Reciprocity in Intergenerational Family Therapy* (New York, Harper and Row, 1973) p2ff

4. Bruce Lackie, "The Family of Origin of Social Workers," *Clinical Social Work Journal*, 1983, Vol II, p321

her a "false self," hiding his/her own true needs for fear that if they would be expressed the family would be strained and could not meet them. Moreover, they are profoundly sensitive to the family's instability. The caregivers as children sustain their family system in which they are raised by taking care of others' needs. They hold the family together by focusing on others and denying themselves. They insure the security of the system they require at the expense of the expression of their personal concerns. In the process, they develop a false self, one compliant, and the other focused. They make others' needs their needs. Their mantra becomes "I help therefore I need no help and in needing no help of my own I find my security, but in order to maintain my security and sense of identity, I must find those who need my help."

In all of the above profiles, the caregiver is essentially a sensitive person, one who is deeply affected by his/her family's needs and vulnerabilities. He/she takes on the responsibility to hold it together at the expense of self. And yet to the extent the caregiver is motivated by these family of origin issues, he/she will not become mature in his/her role. In fact for the caregiver to in the end heal the conflicts that led him/her into his/her vocational choice, he/she will have to fail in his/her role. It is only in failing in one's role that one can come to see his/her efforts as an ultimately unsatisfying way to deal with business that was part of childhood and now needs to be passed over. Typically that failure will occur in the context of the caregiver feeling him/herself burned out or when he/she becomes depressed or simply reactive in his/her role. While others may define the caregiver as having a problem, in fact the response is part of a solution. Given time and attention, he/she will readjust his/her life and claim what is his/her real truth and need. At times he/she will continue to do the work of caregiving with a new focus or better boundaries, or perhaps provide care in a way that feels less driven and more satisfying to the person he/she truly is. At times he/she will let go of the role and choose another context to express his/her vocational choice, say focus one's rabbinate on teaching rather than caregiving. At time he/she may change his/

her vocation altogether.[5]

It is important to note here that having a personal agenda in caregiving is not a bad thing. It is commonplace. In fact virtually all vocational decisions from becoming a plumber to a physician are influenced by psychic needs. Rather our discussion is an attempt for us as caregivers to demystify our interest in this work and call it for the truth that it is, not a heroic gesture that puts us "above" our profit-seeking neighbor but a response to our needs. The humility that engenders, I suspect, is a good thing for caregivers, though not a pill easy to swallow. I surely did not relish Murray's comment to me in the story with which we began the chapter. And yet over time seeing my caregiving as my need freed me from the grandiosity with all its self-judgment. Accepting my work as my need, I could more readily laugh at myself and embrace criticism and learn. Gradually I grew to have less drivenness and better balance. Yes, I still have a need to be needed, but I am better able to get those needs met in other contexts and to make my caregiving an expression of a more authentic self-need, the desire to see others relieved of their suffering. Coming to recognize my own agenda helped me shift its focus from my vocation to my personal life. With that I could keep better boundaries, make better spiritual assessments, and yes at times, when it was in the patient's best interest say "no" to an unhelpful request.

Our tradition makes clear the truth that those who are truly "called" to their mission are not seeking it. On the contrary, they in most cases would have preferred to not pursue it at all. Look at the Biblical characters of Moses and Jeremiah as examples. In the case of Moses, God had to entreat him to accept his role to free the Israelites from bondage. Even then Moses refused to accept the spokesperson's role deferring in the end to his brother Aaron. Jeremiah at first declined God's call for him to prophesize to God's people. Those who were called to historic leadership of the Jewish people were inevitably the least likely to expect their call. From David, the alone shepherd, to Rabbi Akiva, who as an adult was yet uneducated, the story of Jewish leadership is a story of persons

---

5. Allen Wheelis, *The Quest for Identity*, p246

whose call came to them as a surprise. They were not looking for it. They had no need to be needed or if they did it was acted out in other venues. And yet that very attitude made them most worthy of their call. It was precisely because it was clear their leadership was not about the pursuit of ego that they had the right stuff to lead others and with the others' best interest in mind.

As caregivers we need to realize that our best efforts will likely come when we feel least driven to our work. To the extent that our caregiving as rabbi, chaplain, or other provider of emotional/ spiritual support feels compelling we might wonder about its purity. The more we are driven to our work, no matter how sacred, the more we need to suspect it is a work of the ego, our ego. As we mature in our role and get our personal needs met elsewhere we do in fact become less driven to *hesed*. Instead we choose where and how much we can extend ourselves to others. In making choices we can believe we are truly responding to the others and drawing our satisfaction in improving their circumstances.

Judaism refers to the *mitzvah* performed with the highest degree of purity of motivation as a *mitzvah* done *lishma*, for its own sake, that is, done simply to fulfill the command of the Divine. And even though the Talmud taught "A person should forever do *mitzvot* even not *lishma*, for from not *lishma* he/she will eventually come to perform them *lishma*"[6], that does not make intentionality irrelevant to the holy act. A great rabbinic figure was once asked what he could possibly have to repent for when the Day of Atonement came, after all his life was totally immersed in study and good deeds. He responded by pointing to the purity of his actions and said that he had much to improve in making his *mitzvot* more truly *lishma*, more truly motivated solely to do God's will.

The call to intentionality in the arena of caregiving is not only about understanding why we chose for our vocation a focus on *hesed*. The call to intentionality challenges us to look at each pastoral encounter and explore the feelings that encounter engenders in us. So much of the work of Clinical Pastoral Education is helping students come to a heightened level of self-awareness. We learn

---

6. Talmud Jerusalem, Chagigah 1:5

to recognize the dynamics the experience of being with another in the intimacy of a conversation is causing in us. In the language of psychology, we call the feelings another causes in us transference. If we are the provider of care in the encounter, we call it counter-transference. Just think for a moment, have you ever been with another person and felt an instantaneous attraction, or perhaps repulsion? You may wonder why you feel so strongly toward him/her. You may want to attribute your positive or negative regard as a response to who he/she is. But on reflection you come to realize that you really don't know him/her. And even if you did perceive him/her correctly, you still wonder why should it have such a strong impact on you.

In caregiving encounters, those kinds of reactions to persons occur all the time. A chaplain, a man in his twenties, may visit a sixty-year-old woman and without hardly knowing her begin to see her a wonderful person, caring, selfless, devoted to family. In truth she may have lived a life wrapped up in herself and been mean-spirited to her husband. That however is not the story the chaplain will hear. Without knowing it he saw his grandmother in this woman, and engaged her out of an image more true to his life story than her reality. He may have sat at the bedside with the woman for twenty minutes yet he never really met her. Instead he engaged the image of his grandmother she represented. Or take the case of a woman chaplain who visited with a woman of similar age to her mother and with a similar outspokenness. The chaplain may have a visceral negative reaction to the woman patient. Unless the chaplain is called to consciousness, she will not likely realize that her negative feelings toward the patient do not belong to the patient but to her mother. It was her mother that she was reacting to as she conversed with the patient of similar age to her mother and with similar characteristics. Yet this woman, the patient, did not earn the negative response. It will only be when the chaplain comes to the awareness of the counter-transference operating in her relationship with the patient that she can let go of it and be free enough to meet the patient for the patient's self and care for her in the way she needs.

To come to consciousness of the stuff we bring into our pastoral encounters we need supervision. To be unconscious is just that. Without supervision we may never realize when we have engaged someone in the guise of providing care and reacted not to him/her but to someone he/she may represent to us. A core element of Clinical Pastoral Education is the supervision one receives from peers and supervisor on one's clinical care. It is a context to recognizing the transferences and counter-transferences operating in our visits. Even professionals in the field of caregiving, those certified in the work, continue to need supervision, from peers or perhaps senior professionals, to review their work and explore the self-issues that arise in relationship to patients.

Whether we are motivated by a desire to do the *mitzvah* of providing care with the highest degree of *lishma* or whether we are motivated by the professional expectation that we be fully available to the hurting other to offer the most authentic meeting possible, knowing thyself is a critical component of the work of effective caregiving. In most of this book, we discussed the concepts and skills associated with creating healing relationships. To be sure, skills matter. As one wise person once noted, "Counter-transference flourishes in the absence of skills." And yet skills alone are not enough. We must be vigilant in identifying our values, our prejudices, our likes and our dislikes. We must come to recognize where we become reactive out of our own self-story to the dynamics of others. We must invite the supervision of others to help us uncover unconscious transferential feelings that cause us to either care too much or too little for the one hurting.

Caregiving is a work of love. Its root in Jewish tradition emerges out of the commandment "Love thy neighbor as thyself".[7] Like love, it is always in need of refinement. Just as we can never claim we love our spouses or our children perfectly and we are forever challenged to become more loving in relationship with them, so too in caring for others we are forever challenged to deeper and more complete expressions of love. In the pages of this book, we have outlined the holy and at times daunting call to *hesed* in the

7. Leviticus 19:18

forms of *bikur cholim* and *nichum aveilim*. Excellence is the work of a lifetime, never complete. We are forever in process to become more effective. We are agents of healing. Our imperative is to greater authenticity in cultivating a sacred intimacy. And why should that be surprising? After all our initiative is cast in the shadow of the Divine. It is in God's ways that we are walking. May we merit through our care to evidence God's love in the way God wants it known to God's children and in the way the suffering children need to know it in their lives.

Index

52964753R00093

Made in the USA
Middletown, DE
23 November 2017